MW01235499

THE FIBRОМYALGIA REPORT

Blowing the whistle on
chronic fatigue syndrome & fibromyalgia from the clinic

by: Pamela Ross, MMS, PA-C

Published by:
The Institute For Wellbeing
www.instituteforwellbeing.com

ISBN 978-0-9850110-2-4

Printed in the United States of America

The theories, suggestions and ideas contained in this book are not intended to act as a substitute for consulting with your physician and obtaining medical supervision as to any activity or suggestion that may affect your health. Neither the author nor the publisher are engaged in rendering professional advice or services to the individual reader. Accordingly, individual readers must assume responsibility for their own actions, safety, and health as neither the publisher nor the author shall be liable or responsible for any loss, injury or damage allegedly arising from any information or suggestions found in this book.

ACKNOWLEDGEMENTS

Thank you to everyone who supported us at
The Institute For Wellbeing

David Hampton
Henri Nammour, MD
Damon Chase, JD
Judge Tom Freeman
Frank Finkbeiner JD
Professor Wallace Duncan
Autumn
Gina
Ciana
Angela
Paula
Heather
Bob Panek

Many special thanks to each and every patient for sharing their journey with us.

I dedicate this book to my mother, Joan.
Her early departure from this life sparked in me a long,
haunting pursuit, searching for a hidden reason
for the cause of certain disease processes
and answers for health and prevention.

"Nothing in life is to be feared. It is only to be understood."
~Marie Curie

TABLE OF CONTENTS

FORWARD

It seems that many people suffering from chronic fatigue and or fibromyalgia have been deeply disappointed by the medical profession. Patients have been shunned, referred to psychiatry, and/or only given advice on how to reduce stress, without any real answers as to what is going on or any *reason* for their chronic state of pain & fatigue.

"No one believes me." This seems to be an affliction that drives deep into the physical, emotional and spiritual well-being of an individual. It seems to be an affliction set apart from other pathologies because of the longstanding consequences like isolation; mostly, because it is invisible, therefore leaving the afflicted left to explain a myriad of adverse symptoms that exist, without a clinical or laboratory finding. It is almost as if their efforts to express themselves fall onto deaf ears.

If this sounds like something you can relate to, then I hope that this book will provide you with information that will assist you in finding your way back to health and to begin living your life to the fullest, as intended. This report reviews the stories and clinical findings for patients suffering from chronic fatigue syndrome and fibromyalgia.

It is also an effort to offer hope to those who are suffering and a reflection that there are those of us in the health care field who believe you and really do care. At the end, we developed the FIBROBUSTERS® protocol that has helped many others and now we want to share it with you.

I. MRS. JONES

Mrs. Jones has an appointment with her doctor to discuss her relentless symptoms, consisting of . . . *"muscle pain, joint pain, back pain, a headache, acid reflux, irritable bowel syndrome and I can't sleep,"* says Mr. Jones.

The doctor says, *"Let's run some tests – come back in a week and we will discuss the results."*

Mrs. Jones returns in a week, anxious to discover what is causing her list of ailments.

The doctor informs her by stating plainly, *"Your tests are all normal."*

Mrs. Jones replies, *"But Doctor, how can that be? My skin hurts, my scalp hurts and it feels like I am walking on glass. I am anxious, depressed and stressed out!"*

The doctor checks for "trigger points." She has 11 out of 18. He says, *"Mrs. Jones, you have fibromyalgia. Here is a set of prescriptions – come back in a month and we will see how you are doing."* At this point, Mrs. Jones is most likely given an anti-depressant such as Prozac; and/or anti-seizure medication, such as Lyrica, which is currently "indicated" for fibromyalgia.

She returns to the clinic in one month, as directed.

5

The doctor says, *"How are we today Mrs. Jones?"*

Mrs. Jones reports, *"Well Doc, I used to be depressed. Now I am very depressed. I have put on 15 pounds, my head feels swollen and I am having suicidal thoughts."*

The doctor says, *"Oh my! These are side effects from the prescriptions – let's give you a different set of prescriptions, instead."*

Mrs. Jones walks away assessing the past month and decides to get a second opinion. So she goes to a new doctor . . . and then another . . . and yet another.

10 years later, Mrs. Jones shows up at my clinic. She is pulling with her a piece of carry on luggage. *"Hi, Mrs. Jones, come on into room 2. What's in the carry-on?"*

"Oh, this?" She looks down at it as if it were attached to her physically in some way. *"These are my medical records."*

"Wow. And what's in the bag you are carrying over your shoulder?"

She leans sideways to let the weight of the bag slide down her arm, *"These are all of my prescriptions and supplements I am taking."*

Mrs. Jones informs me she has been to numerous doctors over the past 10 years in search of a reason for her pain & fatigue. All of her medical records show no sign of any pathology or abnormality. She tells me that her doctors don't know what else they can do for her.

After reviewing her medical history, and listening to her story, Mrs. Jones tells me that, *"it all began after an accident"* . . . 20 years ago.

CAN YOU DIE FROM FIBROMYALGIA?

I was at a local health fair for the clinic when another vendor across the isle from us rose up out of his chair, walked across the isle, leaned over the table, looked me unwaveringly in the eye and asked me, *"What do you do?"*

"We specialize in chronic fatigue and fibromyalgia," I said.
"How do you treat them?" He asked.
"With respect," I said.

He then reached across the table extending his hand for me to shake and introduced himself.

"My best friend died from fibromyalgia," he explained with emotion rippling over his face.
"I am so sorry. What happened?" I asked.
"She overdosed on pain meds."

II. YOU'RE IN GOOD COMPANY

Fibromyalgia has been around for a very long time and you are not alone. Not only that, but you're in good company. Take a look at some famous people presenting with similar symptoms: Florence Nightingale, Charles Darwin, Alfred Nobel and Job. It is believed that they all suffered from symptoms we know of today as Chronic Fatigue Syndrome and/or Fibromyalgia.

Ms. Nightingale became bedridden with debilitating symptoms for the last half of her life. After the war, she went into her room, closed the door and lay in bed. She did not want visitors, for she suffered from invisible symptoms.

"There is no part of my life, upon which I can look back without pain," Florence Nightingale.

Upon returning to England from traveling in South America and the Pacific Islands, Charles Darwin became incapacitated from headaches, heart palpitations and stomach problems.

Alfred Nobel suffered from constant pain, debilitating migraines, "paralyzing" fatigue and chest pain. In Nobel's letters he describes a 30 year search for a diagnosis by physicians in Europe for what he described as, "a pain that will not go away." People thought he was a hypochondriac. He died in 1896, at the age of 63, bitter and depressed.[1]

The most compelling read is the Old Testament Bible story of Job. Job was a good man, wealthy, with 10 children, servants, property and bountiful livestock. Job suffers total disasters, losing his entire family and everything he owns. Then he is plagued by a disease. This is what he has to say:

"And everything I eat makes me sick . . .
There is nowhere I can turn for help.
In trouble like this I need loyal friends. . .
Night after night brings me grief.
When I lie down to sleep, the hours drag;
I toss all night and long for dawn. . .
I give up; I am tired of living.
Leave me alone.
My life makes no sense . . .
There is no relief for my suffering.
At night my bones all ache.
The pain that gnaws me never stops.
I watch how bitterly everyone mocks me.
I am being honest, God. Accept my word.
There is no one else to support what I say.
You have closed their minds to reason;
Don't let them triumph over me now." [2]

III. "IS IT CHRONIC FATIGUE SYNDROME OR FIBROMYALGIA?"

It might be both.

Fibromyalgia today is now a recognized clinical entity causing chronic and disabling pain.   The CDC reported for 2005 that approximately 2% of the population is affected by fibromyalgia; that number means an estimated 5,000,000 people in the USA, alone.

The Centers for Disease Control and Prevention has estimated the number of Americans with chronic fatigue syndrome (CFS) to be 1 to 4 million and states that it is more common in women than men.   They define CFS as follows: debilitating fatigue with at least 4 of the following: malaise after physical exertion, forgetfulness and inability to concentrate, headaches, sore throat, joint pain, swollen lymph nodes, mild fever, muscle aches, and unexplained muscle weakness.[5, 6]   Not all researchers agree with the criterion defined by the CDC that symptoms must persist more than six months before a diagnosis can be made.

Since 1950, CFS/FM has been described outside of the USA as "myalgic encephalomyelitis," meaning muscle pain with brain and spinal cord inflammation. Clinically, it is in the presentation of symptoms that would typically distinguish between the two. However, a patient could have either or both. Many times symptoms overlap and it varies with each patient:

SHARED SYMPTOMS OF CFS & FIBROMYALGIA

Chronic Fatigue
Widespread joint & muscle pain
Night Sweats
Flu-like Symptoms
Low Grade Fever/Chills
Head Aches/Migraines
Chemical Sensitivities
Skin Rashes
Canker Sores
Restless Leg Syndromes
Irritable Bowel Syndrome
Gastroenteritis
Acid Reflux
Unexplained Chest Pain
Shortness of Breath
Anxiety
Depression
Brain Fog
Sleep Disorders
Dizziness
"My skin hurts"
"It feels like I'm walking on glass"

It seems that patients with CFS suffer more intensely from the psychological aspects including deep depression, extreme fatigue, stress and memory impairment. We'll share with you later the differences we found based on lab results between CFS and FM.

More than their differences, the two afflictions share a great deal in common. Along with the debilitating symptoms, our patients share with us stories of tragedy, despair, lost jobs, divorce, and social isolation because of these illnesses. From what we have seen, chronic fatigue and/or fibromyalgia have no boundaries as to male or female, rich or poor.

Typically, the patient shows up bringing with them volumes of medical records, carried in bags and sometimes boxes, loaded with lab reports, MRIs, CAT scans, EKGs, EEGs, . . And, there are no findings - all tests are essentially normal. We go over a long list of meds that the patient has been prescribed by several different practitioners along the way, and then go through a long list of natural supplements that the patient decided on in a way to "self-medicate. The patient explains in detail his or her experience with overall pain, headaches, night sweats, digestive disorders, brain fog, dizziness, sleep problems, anxiety, depression and so much more. Patients tell me they have suffered for years; for some, 30 years! In the meantime, they lost their jobs, their spouses have left and they are socially isolated. Then they go on to explain that no one believes them. Most of our patients seeking help for their condition have been told by health care practitioners that all of their lab tests and diagnostics are normal and so there is nothing more they can do.

Since there is currently no "cure" for CFS or Fibromyalgia, the medical community will treat the symptoms with prescription drugs ranging from pain meds, anti-virals, antibiotics, sleep meds, muscle relaxers, anti-depressants, anti-anxiety meds, anti-histamines, and the list goes on depending on the symptoms.

A BRIEF HISTORY OF FIBROMYALGIA

So it seems that these symptoms have been around for a very long time and now we have a name for it. A quick look at how the term fibromyalgia was coined:

For several centuries, muscle pains have been known as "rheumatism."
Followed by the term, "muscular rheumatism."
1904 – Gowers coined the term, "Fibrositis."
1972 – Smythe laid foundation of the modern, "fibromyalgia syndrome" by describing widespread pain and tender points.
1976 – Name change from "Fibrositis" to "Fibromyalgia."
1981 – The first controlled clinical study validating known symptoms and *"Tender Points."*
1984 – Proposed concept that Fibromyalgia syndrome and other similar conditions are interconnected.[3]
1990 – American College of Rheumatology criteria published, *"Tender Points."* [3]

TRIGGER POINTS – "THAT'S HOW YOU ARE DIAGNOSING ME WITH FIBROMYALGIA?" asked the patient.

In 1990 the American College of Rheumatology published criteria for Fibromyalgia requiring that the patient had a history of chronic widespread pain, both sides of the body, above and below the waist (affecting all 4 quadrants), along with 11 or more of the 18 "tender points" upon examination. According to an article by Harris, the trigger point criteria was originally established for research purposes only with hopes of establishing, once and for all, a formal diagnosis.

Establishment of a formal diagnosis obviously would be backed by research, making it repeatable and one might add, respected. However, what happened is that practitioners began using these criteria in mainstream medicine more or less as *diagnosis of exclusion* for "Fibromyalgia." This means that after they rule out the possibility of any other disease, then it must be "Fibromyalgia."

To date there is no FDA approved diagnostic test or biomarker in order to standardize the definition of Fibromyagia.[4] All we have is "trigger points." It is believed that this series of events is what has led to the many misconceptions about fibromyalgia.

TRIGGER POINTS 1-18 - all are bilateral

1 and 2:
Low Cervical C5-C7

3 and 4:
Second Rib 2nd costochondral space

5 and 6:
Greater Trochanter Posterior to the trochanteric prominence

7 and 8:
Knees Medial fat pad proximal to the joint line

9 and 10:
Occiput Suboccipital muscle insertions

11 and 12:
Trapezius Midpoint of upper border.

13 and 14:
Supraspinatus Above the scapular spine

15 and 16:
Elbows Lateral Epincondyle

17 and 18:
Gluteals Upper, outer quadrants in the anterior fold of muscle.

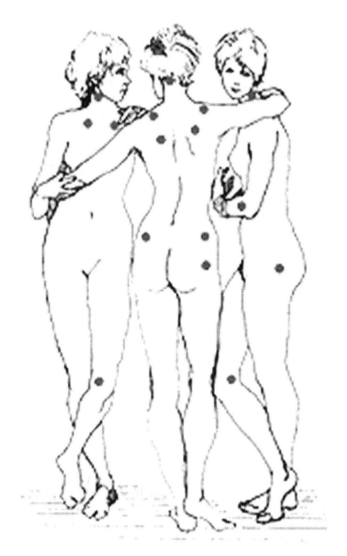

The Three Graces
Baron Jean Baptiste Regnaut
1973

IV. "IT ALL STARTED AFTER THE ACCIDENT"

"It all started after the accident." We hear this many times with our patients; stories of accidents, trauma and extreme stress . . . *"and then the symptoms set in."*

Let's take a look at what happens to us during trauma or stress: According to Deitch, MD, during extreme stress or shock, the body decreases blood flow to the intestines, thereby ensuring critical blood flow to the heart and brain. Meanwhile, the decreased blood flow to the gut causes injury to these tissues. Whether it is minimal or massive, there is some loss of function to the gut barrier. Now we have an opportunity for what most people know as, "leaky gut."
You just lost your filter.

MULTIPLE ORGAN DYSFUNCTION SYNDROME

Mr. Jones, while crossing a busy intersection on foot, was struck by a car. He was taken to the trauma unit where his organs started shutting down one by one. He passed on, not because of broken bones, but because of "multiple organ dysfunction syndrome."

The theory holds that as blood was diverted away from the GI tract to the heart and brain to keep him alive, the loss of blood flow caused injury to the GI lining, allowing pathogens to cross over into circulating blood where they were unwittingly carried to organs and causing damage.

Stress or trauma that causes even small increases in gut permeability will introduce the body to unwanted pathogens. It's these pathogens that cause pain and fatigue at the minimum, with the possibility of leading to damaged organs such as thyroid, lungs and kidneys.

"Considering the normal gut contains enough bacteria and endotoxins to kill the host thousands of times over. We reasoned that even small increases in gut permeability have profound physiological consequences" said Edwin A. Deitch, MD professor and chair of the Department of Surgery at UMDNJ New Jersey Medical School.[48]

BORDER PATROL

We come into contact with infectious pathogens daily. We are generally equipped to marshall such a defense which prevents antigens from crossing over into the body – or, crossing the border, if you will.

Imagine this: a long tube, starting with entry into your nose, leading to the sinuses, which empties into the back of the throat, into the lungs or into the stomach, continuing through the small intestines, large intestines and out the back door. This long tube with an entry and an exit is "outside the body." Anything that passes through this tube is now "inside the body."

Mast cells are one type of immune cell that lines the sinuses, throat, respiratory tract, stomach, intestines, blood

18

vessels, nerves, the skin, and GI tract. Think of them as "border patrol" between the environment and any entryway into your body.

One well known immune response to an antigen trying to cross the border, (to get inside the body) is the release of histamine, primarily causing inflammation. Histamine is released from mast cells in the GI tract in an immune response activated by the antigen or by complement fragments from an antibody (IgM and IgG).

Antibody production to an antigen is a normal immune response. Antibody production activates complement; and complement fragments stimulate mast cells to release histamine. Histamine then activates NMDA receptors in the brain and can cause over excitation of the central nervous system leading to symptoms such as anxiety, stress, insomnia and agitation.

In the end, histamine is a neurotransmitter found abundantly in the central nervous system. The effects of histamine on the brain influence behavior, biological rhythms, body weight, energy metabolism, body temperature, fluid balance, stress and reproduction. More information on histamine and histamine receptors is found in Section XIV. You will also see later in this book that antibody production to combat antigens (anything foreign, like viruses or bacteria) causes inflammation and tissue damage.

19

ENDOTOXINS

According to T.S. Wiley's book, "Lights Out", there is an average of 4 pounds of bacteria in your gut. It is suggested that the number of bacteria rises during the day. These bacteria give off "endotoxins" (bacterial excretions) that eventually activate your immune system causing you to sleep and thus lowering the number of bacteria. If you can't sleep, the endotoxins build and begin to kill off endothelial cells (cells that line the GI tract).

National Geographic News published a most intriguing article entitled, "Bugs in Our Gut Make Us More Than Human," by Mason Inman. The following is an excerpt from this article dated June 1, 2006:

"The ever present armies of microbes in your digestive tract are so essential to your survival, a new study says, that you might consider yourself a super-organism—human plus microbes equals you. . . These hordes of "gut bugs" perform digestive duties that the human body alone cannot, according to the first ever comprehensive study of these microbes' genes. . . The study maps the genes of the estimated 500 or more species that live inside us. . . . About a quarter of these genes appear to belong to unknown species. Our bodies carry ten times more microbial cells than human cells, and these microbes collectively contain at least a hundred times the number of genes in the human genome."

THE GUT - A VIRAL RESERVOIR

Research at UC Davis found that while HIV therapy is successful in reducing the viral count and increasing T-cell count in the peripheral blood, this is not so in the gut mucosa. A three year study reveals that HIV continues to replicate in the gut mucosa at the same time that blood work shows the effectiveness of antiviral therapy.

A quote from Satya Dandekar, professor and chair of the Department of Medical Microbiology and Immunology at UC Davis Health System and senior author of the study, "The real battle between the virus and exposed individuals is happening in the gut immediately after viral infection," she said. "We need to be focusing our efforts on improving treatment of gut mucosa, where massive destruction of immune cells is occurring.

Gut-associated lymphoid tissue accounts for 70 percent of the body's immune system. Restoring its function is crucial to ridding the body of the virus."

She goes on to say, "We found a substantial delay in the time that it takes to restore the gut mucosal immune system in those with chronic infections," Dandekar said. "In these patients the gut is acting as a viral reservoir that keeps us from ridding patients of the virus."[32]

V. COULD IT BE A VIRUS?

First of all, know that viruses are everywhere. They are found in the soil, in the air, on doorknobs, countertops, dishes, towels and more. While some viruses are airborne, others are transmitted through human contact.

Viruses that enter through the nose or mouth, will replicate in the sinuses, back of the throat, or in the gut, initially giving rise to moderate symptoms like a stuffy nose, sore throat and/or upset stomach. If these viruses have the opportunity to multiply in the lymph tissue of the small intestine from where they are able to pass into the regional lymph nodes, this will give rise to a viremia (virus in the blood) with the ability to spread into tissues such as liver, spleen, bone marrow and distal lymph nodes.

Once you are exposed to certain viruses, they are with you for life. They will lie dormant until there is an opportunity, through stress or injury (which creates a point of entry) creating an immune response which will manifest physically in a wide range of symptoms from mild discomfort to an all out seizure.

AN EXOTIC VIRUS
Over the years, there have been reports of outbreaks around the world of chronic- fatigue-like illnesses. According to a recent article in the Wall Street Journal, outbreaks at a Los Angeles hospital in 1934 and a later outbreak at a

British hospital in 1955 were reported by physicians to be caused by a version of the polio virus (enterovirus family).

In March 2011, The Wall Street Journal did a series of articles based on the discovery of the XMRV retrovirus in people with chronic fatigue (this virus was earlier found in prostate tumors). This new information turned up the volume amongst scientists and advisory committees around the globe. It escalated into a ban on blood donations from people with chronic fatigue syndrome out of concern over the findings of this new retrovirus.

Meanwhile, the CDC (Center for Disease Control) reported that it could not duplicate findings for XMRV amongst people with chronic fatigue syndrome.

At least be reassured that there are hundreds of scientists around the globe at work, making enormous efforts to identify the cause of both afflictions.

COMMON VIRUSES

We were looking for viruses, too – however, not the exotic kind – only more common ones that most people have already been in contact with such as Herpes 1-6, Parvo, Enteroviruses and Adenovirus. We found that our patients were making greater than normal amounts of antibodies to these viruses.

Keep in mind that we have all been exposed to most of these viruses and that antibody production is a normal immune response. Generally, we pick up many of these viruses as children and create immunity to them. Typical presentation of a childhood virus is fever, rash, maybe an episode of GI upset, fatigue, and then it's over. So, as you enter into this world, come into contact with people, and begin exploring all that life presents to you, it would be possible to pick up one or two viruses at a time, maybe more, who knows. Maybe you don't even remember. The problem is, they stay with you for life. They hide out in tissue. Add a little trauma or stress, overwhelming the immune system and this gives these viruses an opportunity to come out and wreak havoc – possibly 3 or more of them at a time.

Chronic fatigue and fibromyalgia have been associated with the Epstein Barr Virus (EBV) and other herpes viruses, as well as enteroviruses and others. Virology, the study of viruses, is quite complex and extensive as there are so many. One way to classify the many viruses is by the host cell they infect. For example there are animal viruses, plant viruses, and viruses that infect bacteria and mold. We will look at viruses that are common to the human host.

The enteroviruses are probably the most interesting. They consist of Coxsackie A & B, Echovirus and Polio. This particular family of viruses is where we found a difference between chronic fatigue syndrome and fibromyalgia in our patients. It seemed that patients with symptoms of chronic fatigue syndrome and also suffering more from extreme depression, along with other psychological aspects, were making antibodies to coxsackie A & B and echovirus.

THE VIRAL PANEL
Common viruses and associated symptoms:

Herpes 1&2	Herpes 3 (Varicella Zoster)	Herpes 4 (Epstein Barr)	Herpes 5 (Cytomegalovirus)
cold sores	chicken pox	mononucleosis	low grade fever
fever blisters	shingles	low grade fever	swollen lymph
low grade fever	trigeminal neuralgia	sore throat	sore throat
swollen lymph	myelitis	Oral hairy leukoplakia (viral replication on tongue)	joint stiffness
encephalitis	post-herpetic neuralgia		difficulty swallowing
seizures	Ramsey Hunt Syndrome	Throat cancer	pneumonia
depression	Bell's Palsey	joint stiffness	GI distress
fatigue	fatigue	swollen lymph	vision problems
		enlarge spleen	hearing problems
		weakness	
		weight loss	lack of coordination
		lymphoma	
		seizures	seizures
		depression	weakness
		fatigue	discomfort
			weight loss
			depression
			fatigue

Continued –
Common viruses and associated symptoms:

Herpes 6 (Roseola)	Parvo B-19	Coxsackie & Echo (enteroviruses)	Adenovirus
low grade fever	low grade fever	low grade fever	low grade fever
rash	rash	rash	swollen lymph
swollen lymph	swollen lymph	swollen lymph	sore throat
myocarditis	joint pain	joint pain	headache
seizures	myocarditis	muscle pain	congestion
depression	anemia	myocarditis	shortness of breath
fatigue	fatigue	pericarditis	
		myelitis	pneumonia
		meningitis	GI distress
		orchitis	dysuria
		shortness of breath	depression
			fatigue
		cough	
		weakness	
		seizures	
		anxiety	
		depression	
		fatigue	

The following is a recent case study in JAAPA *(Journal of the American Academy of Physician Assistants)*:

"IT ALL STARTED AFTER THE ACCIDENT"

A lady showed up at her doctor's office complaining of a headache, fever, nausea, vomiting and discomfort. After some standard testing, which all came back normal, she was diagnosed with an upper respiratory viral infection. She went home.

Her symptoms became worse over the next few days and her headache was not relieved with medication. She had a dizzy spell and decided to go to the ER. While taking her history, she recalled a biking accident 2 weeks earlier which resulted in a cracked helmet. She stated that she continued to ride anyway without difficulty. They ran some more tests, which all came back normal, and diagnosed her with a mild concussion. She went home.

That night, her fever rose and she had another dizzy spell. She woke up with a serious headache and in a state of confusion with memory impairment. She returned to the ER. She was admitted with a diagnosis of viral meningitis. The next day her cerebral spinal fluid was positive for herpes simplex 1. Later, an MRI revealed encephalitis (swelling of the brain). She was discharged many days later with a diagnosis of herpes encephalitis (swelling of the brain because of herpes).

Her recovery took months. She was extremely fatigued and slept most days for the first 6 weeks; after which she became extremely depressed with thoughts of suicide. She still had trouble with her memory. She was prescribed therapy for speech, memory and ability to maintain attention. She was eventually able to return to work; however, she continued to suffer from extreme fatigue in the evenings and persistent stress.

Herpes simplex 1 is the most common cause of random encephalitis in the USA.[47] Primary infection of herpes occurs through a break in the skin or mucous membrane. It then travels up a nerve to a neuron (nerve cell) in the central nervous system where it lies dormant.

In this case, herpes encephalitis is thought to reach the brain by ascending the trigeminal nerve (in the face) or olfactory nerve (in the nose).[47] It is proposed that the virus was able to reach the brain after the biking accident, which would have caused the inflammation, creating a point of entry for the virus that preexisted in the central nervous system.

VI. TOO MANY ANTIBODIES

Again, antibody production to antigens (like viruses) is a normal immune response; however, **antibody production does not control an infection** – it is a signal to reveal what we are trying to get rid of in our system. It is when we make too many antibodies that we begin to display adverse symptoms, like pain and inflammation.

The medical term is **"hypersensitivity reaction"** and it is measured by antibody production found in the blood (IgG). The outcome of too many antibodies can range from mild discomfort to irreversible tissue damage and autoimmune disorders (see chapter VII).

Patients with complaints of fatigue, joint pain, muscle pain, headache, scratchy throat, acid reflux, irritable bowel syndrome, back pain, chest pain, shortness of breath, and "it feels like I'm walking on glass", depression, anxiety and sleep disorders, without any explanation as to why and with otherwise normal lab results, were tested for antibody production to common viruses.

Antibody production activates complement; and complement fragments stimulate mast cells to release histamine. Histamine then activates NMDA receptors in the brain and can cause over excitation of the central nervous system, leading to symptoms such as anxiety, stress, insomnia and agitation.

You will see in this section how the "invisible" symptoms of chronic fatigue syndrome & fibromyalgia match symptoms of chronic viral infections.

More information on herpes 1-6, Parvo, Adeno and Enteroviruses is found near the end of the book.

The following are stories of 3 patients who suffer from chronic fatigue and/or fibromyalgia along with simplified lab findings reflecting over production of antibodies to viruses and also to products of their environment:

SIDE EFFECTS OF BEAUTY – A CASE STUDY

Patient #12: An attractive 49 year old female complains of fatigue, herpes outbreaks, canker sores and a white tongue.

Patient states that she suffers from chronic herpes outbreaks and is looking for relief. She states that her genital region hurts in the same area as from previous outbreaks. She says that her mouth hurts from the canker sores and her tongue is white. She had breast implants 18 years ago. She states mild discomfort in the chest and wonders if they are leaking. She believes her overall condition is from an unidentified autoimmune disorder.

Assessment: No significant findings upon physical exam. Recent lab work from another clinic is unremarkable.

IgG Viral Panel:
Herpes 2
Epstein-Barr
Varicella Zoster
CMV

MRI revealed ruptured intracapsular breast implant.

Comments: This CMV (cytomegalovirus) titer was the highest I have ever seen.   CMV can be sexually transmitted, as it is found in sperm.   Shortly thereafter, she discovers that her spouse was seeing other women.   She separated from her husband and has since had the implant replaced.   Her overall condition is much improved.   The chronic viral infection and outbreaks have subsided.

Below is partial copy of lab test for pt #12 showing a CMV IgG value of 17.4.   A negative value would be less than 1:

X Cytomegalovirus (CMV) Ab, IgG
   CMV Ab, IgG (Cytomegalovirus)
                                    17.4   High   index   0.0 - 0.8   01
                                                       Negative   <0.9

"THIS IS JUST THE WAY GOD MADE YOU" said the doctor

Patient #15: 26 year old male with CFS/FM, headache, irritable bowel syndrome, acid reflux, abdominal pain, orchitis (swelling of the testes) and pain in left side of chest x 4 years.

History: He was a victim of hurricane Katrina and was exposed to contaminated flood waters. Patient has been suffering from these symptoms of joint and muscle pain, dizziness, fatigue, headaches, IBS, chest pain, stomach pain, testes pain, night sweats, memory problems x 4 years. He does not want prescription medications. He was diagnosed by a doctor with chest and abdominal pain due to "anxiety and acid reflux."

His doctor told him, "All of your tests are great; this is just the way God made you."

Another physician prescribed an anti-inflammatory for a condition which he concluded to be "costochondritis" (inflammation of the cartilage between the ribs) for the "left rib pain" as described by the patient. The patient ended up in the ER with the rib pain and the physician there told him it was due to anxiety. He was later given Lexapro for the anxiety which subsequently caused tremors and sleep disturbances.

Still suffering from headaches and anxiety the patient could not understand why he felt like he was falling apart. He went to a neurologist for his headaches and after an MRI was told, "stop working out muscles that would irritate the neck."

Some time later, the patient fell and dislocated his shoulder, for which he needed surgery. After surgery the patient experienced extreme stress and heart palpitations at night. He returned to the cardiologist who put him on a halter monitor, performed a stress test and ultrasound. The results revealed no abnormal findings. The physician told him, "Your heart is strong; there is no treatment for these symptoms and try to keep stress levels under control."

A few months later after the surgery he noticed his knees were clicking. Thereafter, all of his joints started to bother him to include wrists, both shoulders, hips, ankles and the biggest source of pain, the spine. He went to a general practitioner who ran a battery of tests to include a complete hormone panel, abdominal CT scan, sleep study, and gluten test. All tests were normal so the physician referred him back to the neurologist for further testing. The neurologist performed a needle nerve conduction test for the left side of his body, more blood work, a lumbar and cervical MRI. According to the physician, the results revealed mild degenerative disk disease and elevated CPK due to exercise. He was told to return in 5 months if there was any change in his condition. He returned for pain radiating into his left arm. An MRI and EKG was done and the results were completely normal.

Still looking for relief, he then went to a naturopath who gave him a detox and supplement regimen in order to heal the gut and reduce inflammation. This plan gave him relief, however, when he returned to his normal solid foods, the pain and problems returned. He has since had colonic sessions which gave relief; accupuncture with short term relief; he tried pilates which exacerbated his symptoms.

The patient was left with the following diagnoses: costochondritis, fibromyalgia, IBS, headache, leaky gut syndrome, degenerative joint disease, orchitis, depression and anxiety. The patient states he has been thrown in many directions and without any real answers. He is mentally drained from it all. He states he does not have any troubling life issues; he has a good life except for all of the debilitating pain. It is difficult for him to understand how at 26 years old he could be experiencing such undue pain and fatigue.

Goal: Patient states he wants to know the reason for his symptoms. He wants to return to the gym and a normal active lifestyle for a healthy 26 year old male.

Assessment: Patient is a body builder. No outstanding clinical findings on exam.

IgG Viral Panel
2 strains of Echovirus
4 strains of Coxsackie virus
Human herpes virus 6.

IgG Environmental Panel

Orange	Trichophyton
Calcium Propionate	Nickel chloride
Apple	Cola
Garlic	FD&C Yellow #10
BHA	Lead

Comments:

1.) Coxsackie and Echovirus are part of the Enterovirus family. Coxsackie has its own 2 strains: A and B. Both can cause myocarditis, which is inflammation of the heart tissue due to infection. It is very painful (feels like a heart attack) and a probable cause of the patient's "rib pain" and upper left abdominal pain. A definitive diagnosis would require a heart biopsy.

2.) Echovirus was probably a result of contaminated waters due to hurricane Katrina. It is the most reasonable cause for the gastrointestinal symptoms since this virus lives in the GI tract. As well, exposure to this particular virus sets up a playground for other opportunistic infections. Again, this virus also is a cause for myocarditis and this virus also causes orchitis.

82% of stomach biopsy samples from 165 chronic fatigue syndrome patients were positive for enterovirus infections. *Chia JK. Chronic fatigue syndrome is associated with chronic enterovirus infection of the stomach. Journal of Clinical Pathology. 2008. Jan. 61 (1) 43-38.*

3.) Human Herpes virus 6 is part of the Herpes family of viruses which to date consist of 8 different strains. In addition, HHV-6 has 2 strains of its own: A and B. A is capable of infecting nerve cells. B is implicated again, in myocarditis.

4.) TRICHOPHYTON is found in showers and other damp floors. It is the fungus found in athlete's foot.

5.) CALCIUM PROPIONATE is found in anti-fungal medication. So not only does the patient suffer from trichophyton, but also is reacting adversely to the medication which was meant to treat the fungus in the first place. Again, making antibodies to this would be indicative of an already overwhelmed immune system.

6.) NICKEL is one of the most common causes of skin allergies. Nickel has the ability to pass through the skin at the hair follicle and sweat ducts. It can be found in eye glass frames, jewelry and more.

7.) It is also reasonable to assume that the headaches are due to an onslaught of immune activity causing pain and inflammation.

An overwhelmed immune system may certainly lead to an exhaustion of nutrient resources to include glycogen, oxygen, enzymes, minerals and essential vitamins. Add to that any malabsorption due to irritable bowel syndrome.

It is also of interest to note that this patient suffered from severe anxiety and sleep disturbance after his shoulder surgery. This may not be coincidence as surgery basically induces stress and trauma. It appears that his immune system is already overwhelmed as evidenced by the overproduction of antibodies. Another natural immune response to consider is histamine release, which not only causes inflammation, but also anxiety.

At the same time, this patient's environment now has greater influence, by an increase in sensitivity naturally due to the effect of inflammatory factors (cytokines) and histamine secreted by an overwhelmed immune system; which may be responsible for the following symptoms: night sweats, chronic pain, fatigue, leaky gut, headaches, depression, anxiety, sleep disorders and memory problems. Add to that the symptoms from viral infection: chest pain, shortness of breath, orchitis (swelling of the testes caused by echovirus) and overall discomfort.

"METHADONE DIDN'T WORK," said the patient

Patient #13: 37 year old male with fibromyalgia x 9 years.

HISTORY: Patient states he has been sick since high school (20+ years).   His symptoms include: night sweats, headaches, shortness of breath, "heart hearts," sore throat, difficulty swallowing, acid reflux, IBS, muscle and joint pain, feet hurt, dizziness, depression, brain fog, trouble sleeping, sensitive to sound and light, restless leg syndrome and Reynaud's syndrome (painful spasms of the blood vessels).   He has a wife and beautiful children age 2 and 5 years old.   He states It is difficult to enjoy them due to his symptoms.

GOAL: The patient wants to get well.   He wants to discontinue his list of prescription medications.   He would like to be able to enjoy his family.

ASSESSMENT: Over the course of a couple of years he was prescribed by his physician the following prescriptions: Buproprion (anti-depressant), Ablilify (add on treatment for depression), Lisinopril (for high blood pressure) Oxycodone (for severe pain; side effect: impairs thinking and reactions, habit forming), Methadone (for pain syndrome, traditionally used for heroine withdrawal; side effect: confusion, habit forming).   The patient states, "Methadone didn't work."

Soma (muscle relaxer; side effect: impairs thinking, habit forming). As stated in the records, the patient states that these meds do not relieve the pain. The patient was pleasant, yet had no expression or emotion, no eye contact, and spoke using short sentences.

IgG viral panel
6 strains of coxsackie virus
Epstein Barr virus
HSV 1 and 2
Parvovirus B-19
Varicella-Zoster
Cytomegalovirus
Adenovirus

Tick panel
1 band of Lyme *(see chapter XI)*

IgG Environmental Panel

Rhizopus stolonifer	Vinyl chloride
Egg yolk	Carmine/cochineal
White potato	Rhizopus nigricans
Black pepper	Barium sulfate
Corn sugar	

Comments:
1.) Coxsackie is the most likely cause of the "heart pain," as it can cause myocarditis (inflammation of the heart). As well, any virus could infect the brain and spinal cord and cause dangerous inflammation. This inflammation can

produce a wide range of symptoms to include: sensitivity to light and sound, fever, headache, and confusion.

2.) Epstein Barr is repeatedly associated with auto-immunity in many journal articles.

3.) Varicella zoster infects nerves and is very painful. It may (or may not) surface in a blistering of the skin along the nerve path.

4.) The symptoms of CMV (cytomegalovirus) infection are similar to those of mononucleosis: fatigue, general discomfort, uneasiness, ill feeling, joint stiffness, loss of appetite, muscle aches or joint pain, night sweats, prolonged fever, sore throat, swelling of the lymph nodes, weakness and weight loss. CMV could also cause CNS symptoms such as sensitivity to light and sound.

5.) Adenovirus affects linings of the lungs and intestinal tract. It is a probable cause for the shortness of breath and attributing to irritable bowel syndrome.

6.) 1 band of Lyme – an indication that his immune system is possibly over responsive?

7.) Rhizopus nigricans and nigricans (mold) – an indication that he is probably becoming sensitive to his environment.

8.) Vinyl Chloride is found in aerosol sprays, as in room deodorizers – possibly used to mask the smell of mold.

Patient states the house is sprayed daily, sometimes more than once.

9.) Corn sugar – patient admits that the use of methadone causes sugar cravings. This test indicates that he has now developed antibodies to sugar.

VII. "IS IT FIBROMYALGIA OR LUPUS?"

When talking with many fibromyalgia patients, lupus, at some point enters the conversation. *"My symptoms come and go in cycles; and it's either from the fibromyalgia or the Lupus."*

Many patients who are diagnosed with lupus have never been told what it is. First of all, it is an auto immune disorder meaning that you are making antibodies to yourself as if your immune system doesn't recognize you. . If your immune system does not recognize your own DNA, it will mount a defense against it by making antibodies and try to get rid of it. This is lupus.

How did this happen? A virus replicates itself using your DNA. The number of viral particles increases to a point where the cell breaks open and the contents of the cell spills into the serum. The spill not only includes millions of replicated viral particles, but also the cells own organelles, including your DNA, which was used by the virus to replicate itself, which now your body doesn't recognize. Could it be that the viral replication process altered your DNA to the point where your immune system doesn't recognize it anymore?

In any event, this now floating immune complex of DNA + antibody, trying to make its way out of the body, will likely become lodged in the joints, kidneys and/or lungs causing significant inflammation and damage.

In a review of literature, entitled, "Viral Infection Can Induce the Production of Autoantibodies," by Barzilai and Ram, they focus on recent findings that associate Epstein Barr and Cytomegalovirus to various autoimmune disorders.

It is suggested that Epstein Barr is associated with lupus, multiple sclerosis, Sjogren's syndrome, autoimmune thyroiditis, autoimmune hepatitis and Kawasaki disease.

It is suggested that Cytomegalovirus is associated with anti phospholipid syndrome, systemic sclerosis, inflammatory bowel disease and diabetes mellitus.[33]

The authors make it clear that further investigation into these associations is needed; as there are steps to developing an autoimmune disorder.   First, there is a likely genetic component; second there is an environmental factor (in this case, a virus) that would allow activation of the genetic component.[19]

Could it be that a chronic viral infection triggers the genetic expression for autoimmune disorders?

Below is table of *autoimmune diseases* in correspondence with tissues unrecognized by the immune system:

AUTOIMMUNE DISEASES:

NAME OF DISEASE	UNRECOGNIZED TISSUE
Addison's disease	Adrenal glands
Hemolytic Anemia	Red blood cells
Celiac	Gut
Crohn's Disease	Gut
Goodpasture's Syndrome	Kidney & Lungs
Grave's Disease	Thyroid
Hashimoto's Thyroiditis	Thyroid
Idiopathic Thrombo-cytopenia Purpura	Platelets
Diabetes mellitus	Pancreatic beta cells
Lupus	DNA, Platelets
Multiple Sclerosis	Brain & Spinal Cord
Myasthenia Gravis	nerve/muscle synapses
Pemphigus Vulgaris	Skin
Pernicious Anemia	Gastric Parietal Cells
Post-strep Glomerulonephritis	Kidneys
Psoriasis	Skin
Rheumatoid Arthritis	Connective tissue
Scleroderma	Heart, Lungs, Gut, Kidneys
Sjogren's Syndrome	Liver, Kidney, Brain, Thyroid, Salivary Glands
Spontaneous Infertility	Sperm

VIII. GUT/BRAIN CONNECTION

Remember Mrs. Jones with complaints of fatigue, *muscle pain, joint pain, a headache, acid reflux, irritable bowel syndrome, back pain, sleep problems, anxiety and depression*; and the doctor who could not find anything wrong with her; so he gave her an anti-depressant (to increase serotonin) and/or Lyrica (anti-seizure medication)?

The gut is also referred to as the "Enteric Nervous System," as it contains more than 100 million neurons. The gut is connected to the brain mainly by the vagus nerve.

According to a recent article in Scientific America, "90% of fibers from the vagus nerve carry information *to* the brain and not the other way around."[53, 54]

Serotonin – made in the Gut and sent to the brain
Serotonin   is primarily made by enterochromaffin cells in the **GUT**. Serotonin is released in response to food. It then passes through the GI membrane and into the blood where it is picked up by platelets and then dropped off onto other cells with serotonin receptors.

Serotonin receptors in the brain are primarily located in the limbic system.[34]   Note that this is where emotions are controlled – as serotonin from the gut is known for impulse control in the brain.

Anti-depressants increase serotonin levels and are written as a prescription for panic disorder, OCD (obsessive compulsive disorder) and social anxiety disorder.

It is believed by many that increasing serotonin levels will alleviate anxiety and depression.   Or does it?   The following is an excerpt from T.S. Wiley's, "Lights Out":   *"When a rat is caught in the open by a predator, the serotonin rises in his brain and he freezes, apparently paralyzed by fear. As nature would have it, by freezing in suspended animation, he is evading all the predators whose vision depends on motion for detection."*[49]

The following is a list of side effects and precautions for anti-depressants taken from a physician prescribing reference:

Side effects: *CNS stimulation (anxiety, nervousness, insomnia) GI upset, sexual dysfunction, somnolence, decreased libido, anorexia, weight loss, agitation, tremor, dry mouth, sweating, motor impairment, platelet dysfunction, hyper/hypo glycemia.*

Here is a really brief explanation of some of the negative side-effects of serotonin re-uptake inhibitors:

Low libido: sexual dysfunction from chronic high serotonin causing imbalance in dopamine.

Weight gain: chronic high serotonin = chronic high insulin, leading to insulin resistance and fat storage.

Precautions: *Monitor for mania, suicidal tendencies & seizures.*

Serotonin makes melatonin which brings up GABA receptors.

GABA signals cell shut down.

There is a balance between GABA and NMDA;

As GABA increases, so does NMDA.

NMDA receptors are the "On" switch for the cell.

Meanwhile, excessive antibody production to pathogens, like viruses, activates complement, which creates complement fragments, activating mast cells that release histamine, which also activates NMDA.

Therefore, overstimulation of NMDA would create over excitation of the central nervous system, creating symptoms of stress, anxiety, nervousness, insomnia, agitation and tremors.

Too many NMDA receptors "On" at the same time would then cause seizures.

It has been suggested that a disruption in the balance of GABA and NMDA receptors triggers a **seizure** . . .

IX. VIRUSES AND THEIR ROLE IN SEIZURES

An interesting note at this point is that the leading pharmaceutical indicated for fibromyalgia is an anti-seizure medication.

It has been suggested that seizures could be linked to disrupted balances in the transmission of GABA (off switch for cells) and NMDA (on switch for cells).

NMDA is the name of the cell receptor that causes an excitatory response. Over excitation of the NMDA receptor allows for movement of too much calcium into the cell causing damage to the mitochondria and therefore damage to the nerve.

It is this movement of the calcium into the cell, thus lowering the calcium levels outside the cell, that causes the excitation of the nervous system, which, if it goes too far, will end up in a seizure.

One research group has shown that cytotoxic granules, secreted by CD8[+] T cells to kill virus-infected cells, are capable of triggering NMDA over-excitation, resulting in nerve degeneration.[22] Another study shows that T cells are present in significant numbers in brains infected with viruses.[23, 24] Therefore, this mechanism of over-excitation may play a larger role than currently realized.

49

In the clinical setting, it is acute fevers that cause seizures in patients with viral encephalitis.[26] As noted so far, herpes 1,2,4,5,6 and enteroviruses are implicated in seizure activity.

Many viruses, especially those capable of triggering seizures, show a natural affinity for nerves within the limbic structures, especially the hippocampus.[25] The limbic system is interconnected to other areas of the brain and includes the olfactory nerve, giving you sense of smell, and the hippocampus, known for storage of memory. While the limbic system has a diverse set of functions, it is best known for its involvement in motivation and emotional behaviors.

The subject of seizures caused by viruses may seem extreme but it does happen; however, at the other end of extreme, *what if* it explains symptoms that match up with consequences of an over excited nervous system such as sensitive emotions, behavior changes, anxiety and stress?

Viral encephalitis affects approximately 7 people out of 100,000 and carries a high rate of morbidity and mortality. Most patients with viral encephalitis will develop some form of seizure during the infectious process, and of those who survive, less than 20% will develop epilepsy. Several DNA viruses that prefer to live in nerves, including herpes and cytomegalovirus, also commonly cause seizures in infected patients.

Insects transmitting viruses (such as West Nile Virus, Rift Valley Fever, and Yellow Fever), are the leading cause of viral encephalitis in the world today. Between 10% - 35% of these patients will display some type of seizure activity.

Seizures

Seizure disorders are a group of syndromes caused by the misfire of neurons within the CNS (central nervous system). The World Health Organization estimates that epilepsy affects 8 people out of a 1,000. Seizures are the net result of imbalances between excitatory and inhibitory inputs within the brain. These disturbances may occur in a specific brain region which would cause a partial seizure or in the whole cortex which would result in a generalized seizure. [19, 20]

Petit mal seizures are particularly fascinating because it is the term commonly given to a "staring spell" (or looks like someone is daydreaming); most commonly called an "absence seizure." It lasts typically less than 15 seconds. Petit mal seizures occur most commonly in people under age 20, usually in children ages 6 to 12. Typical symptoms may include: no movement, hand fumbling, eye fluttering, unintentional staring episode, full recovery without confusion and no memory of it happening. The person does not fall and is wide awake. Most absence seizures go on for a while without being noticed and may be mistaken for "not paying attention." [21]

51

Sometimes a seizure is related to a temporary condition, such as exposure to drugs, withdrawal from certain drugs, a high fever, or abnormal levels of sodium or glucose in the blood. A seizure may also occur as a result of a stroke or a tumor. If the underlying problem is corrected and the seizures stop, then the person does NOT have epilepsy. [13]

The seizure cascade is complicated. The work discussed here clearly shows that seizures occurring as a result of viral infection may involve several mechanisms occurring at the same time.

X. THE ENVIRONMENTAL PANEL

"Ok, Mrs. Jones, we've covered a lot of territory. Is there anything else that you can think of that you would like to tell me?"

"Well, yes. I wanted to let you know that when I walked into this clinic that I could smell the paint on the walls, I could smell the carpet in here . . . and I was wondering, would you please ask the lady at the front desk not to wear that perfume next time I come in? It's making me sick."

MULTIPLE CHEMICAL SENSITIVITY SYNDROMES

As noted previously, we tested not only for viruses and tick borne illnesses, we also ran an IgG environmental panel. The importance of this test is in identifying items that are creating excessive antibody production. Again, these antibodies are an immune response causing inflammation by the activation of complement; which causes a cascade of other events, such as, activation of mast cells releasing histamine which adversely affects the central nervous system. The test results for each patient were very individual, as would be expected, based on exposure. However, we wanted to share just a few of these test items with you.   We are presenting our findings in a mixed fashion — some of it with recent supporting articles and some right from the lab test itself. [36]

53

ASPARTAME

"In response to "Most Faux Sugars Sweeten Foods Safely" (Dec. 6): The most recent research from Spain shows that aspartame (NutraSweet) ingestion leads to formaldehyde accumulation in organs and tissue. Formaldehyde has been proven to cause gradual damage to the nervous and immune systems and has been shown to cause irreversible genetic damage.

Extremely large numbers of toxicity reactions to aspartame have been reported. Symptoms include seizures, headaches, memory loss, tremors, convulsions, vision loss, nausea, dizziness, confusion, depression, irritability, anxiety attacks, personality changes, heart palpitations, skin diseases, loss of blood sugar control, arthritic symptoms and weight gain."

Source: LA Times newspaper December 13, 1999

"Aspartame/nutrasweet is a compound manufactured from two amino acids, aspartic acid and phenylalanine.

By law, Aspartame must be labeled. People sensitive to Aspartame have complained of dizziness, headaches, high blood pressure, hives, agitation, and menstrual irregularities. There are still some doubts about the safety of Aspartame. If it is stored on shelves for a long period, particularly in warm areas, it will release methanol (wood alcohol), which is toxic, causing permanent blindness and death in high enough doses. Overconsumption of Aspartame can potentially cause headaches, high blood pressure, and behavioral changes, particularly in children.

54

Sources of Exposure: diet soda, breath mints, chewable multivitamins and other medications (check with your pharmacist), instant coffee, chewing gum, fruit-juice-based and fruit-flavored drinks, gelatins, puddings, frozen-stick-type confections, and tea beverages." [36]

MERCURY

According to an article in New Beauty Magazine, Minnesota became the first state to outlaw mercury in cosmetics. Undisclosed amounts of mercury can be found in some mascara, eyeliners and skin-lightening creams. Currently, the U.S. allows up to 65 parts per million of mercury as preservative in eye products. [37, 38]

Heavy metals can displace the active trace minerals of zinc, selenium and magnesium from the biologically active enzymes. Heavy metals have a stronger binding coefficient for the amino acid structure of the enzyme than the trace minerals. When cadmium or mercury or any other heavy metal displaces a trace mineral like zinc or selenium from the enzyme it does not function properly. Electrons are then free to flow undirected throughout the cell and free radical production spins out of control. You could not take enough anti-oxidants to keep up with the free radical production which in turn causes inflammation that now has taken up permanent residency within the tissues.

DIBUTYL PHTHALATE

According to a consumer advocacy organization called the Environmental Working Group, nail polish may lead to adverse health issues for the user. The reason for this is due to two chemicals found in some polishes: dibutyl phthalate and toluene. They have been suspect in causing a wide variety of side effects from headaches to birth defects. The US Cosmetic Toiletry and Fragrance Association insists that, since the FDA has continued allowing these ingredients, that they will not harm nail polish users. Europe, however, has voluntarily banned nail polish that contains DBP.[39, 40]

"Two phthalate esters (butylbenzyl phthalate and di-n-butylphthalate) have been shown to be estrogenic, that is they are capable of acting like estrogens and attaching to estrogen receptors in the cell. Animal experiments show an association between liver cancer and phthalate exposure, but this has not been demonstrated as yet in humans. Exposure is primarily through breathing, eating and contact with eyes and skin.

Sources of Exposure: Diethyl phthalate is used in many cosmetics and personal products including eye shadows, toilet waters, perfumes, other fragrance preparations, hair sprays and nail polish removers . . ." [36]

SOAP

The University of Rochester School of Medicine & Dentistry recently published a study linking soap to obesity. Apparently, a chemical commonly found in soap—phthalates—has been identified as a possible cause of excess fat. Previously, research proved that phthalates were responsible for low testosterone levels; men with low testosterone levels tend to develop abdominal obesity, so the study's authors speculated that phthalates could be the missing link.[41]

"Soap is made from a combination of an animal or vegetable fat with sodium hydroxide. Most soaps contain sodium dodecyl sulfate (SDS), also known as sodium lauryl sulfate (SLS).

Soap is not considered a "cosmetic" and therefore is not affected by the cosmetic labeling laws which require ingredients to be listed. Although a few companies voluntarily disclose their ingredients, most do not . . . The study also warned that deodorant soaps should not be used on infants under six months of age. . . "[36]

Sodium Lauryl Sulfate is a commonly used surfactant in soaps, shampoos, toothpaste and detergents. SLS is synthetically made and mimic estrogen. The use of *some* SLS products is banned in Europe, Central America and the Middle East.

Parabens are widely used as a preservative in cosmetics and pharmaceuticals. Parabens in commercial products are synthetically made and also mimic estrogen.

Phthalates have been found to disrupt the endocrine system as they mimic estrogen.

TOO MUCH ESTROGEN?

Estrogen is a hormone that is found in both men and women. Natural estrogens and chemicals that mimic estrogen attach and activate estrogen receptors. Excess estrogen will result in adverse symptoms. It is questionable whether regulating glands of the body are able to differentiate between natural estrogen and synthetic chemicals that mimic estrogen.

In healthy men, estrogen levels are naturally low and yet balanced by other hormones such as testosterone. If this balance is upset by any increase in estrogen, the result becomes a clinical finding such as breast enlargement and reduced sperm count and motility.

In women, estrogen levels are naturally higher than in men and yet balanced by progesterone and testosterone. Excessive estrogen levels will result in adverse symptoms.

This following list contains symptoms and conditions associated with estrogen dominance from John Lee MD: [43]

Breast cancer
Cervical dysplasia
Depression
Increase in fat
Fatigue
Fibrocystic breast tissue
Brain Fog
Hair loss
Headaches
Low blood sugar
Increased blood clotting
Infertility
Irregular menstruation
Insomnia
Memory loss
Mood swings
Polycystic ovaries
PMS
Prostate cancer
Uterine fibroids
Uterine cancer

Concern has been voiced by some researchers and consumer watchdog organizations that parabens, sulfates and phthalates included in cosmetics may disrupt the endocrine system when applied to the skin.

XI. "DO I HAVE LYME DISEASE?"
asked the patient

Many patients report having been bitten by a bug and remember feeling sick thereafter. Often times they have been tested for tick borne illnesses and the results come back inconclusive. It is especially frustrating when all other labs are normal, too, as the patient is trying to find an answer for the onset of "invisible symptoms." Nevertheless, the possibility of a tick borne illness or illness from other pests can not be overlooked. Symptoms may masquerade as CFS/FM. Let your health care practitioner know if you have been bitten by a bug. Here are a few possibilities of diseases transmitted by insect bites:

babesia – Spread through the saliva of a tick when it bites. Babesiosis is caused by a parasite in the blood. Babesia is similar in effect to Plasmodium falciparum, the causative agent of malaria. Symptoms of Babesiosis: fatigue, malaise, myalgia, arthralgia, chills, and fever. This may also cause hemolytic anemia.

b. burgdorferi – spread through tick bites, it is a gram negative spirochete bacteria – the cause of Lyme disease.
Symptoms of Lyme: fatigue, headache, fever, rash, (looks like a bullseye). Without early intervention, symptoms may lead to joint pain, heart problems and central nervous system disorders.

bartonella – spread by flies, mosquitoes and fleas, most of the time transmitted to humans through an animal scratch or bite – it is a gram negative intracellular bacteria associated with Cat Scratch Disease. Symptoms of Bartonellosis: swollen lymph, fatigue, endocarditis.

ehrlichia – spread through ticks, it is an intracellular bacteria. Patients diagnosed with Ehrlichia should also be tested for Lyme disease due to the fact that co-infections have been documented in several patients. It is transmitted in part by the SAME TICKS that carry Lyme disease. Symptoms of Ehrilichiosis: fatigue, high fever, malaise, headache, myalgia, sweats, and nausea.

rickettsia – spread by ticks, fleas, mites and lice – it is a gram-negative, intracellular bacteria. Associated with Rocky Mountain Spotted Fever. Symptoms: headache, fever, abdominal pain, vomiting and muscle pain, with or without the distinctive rash. Rocky Mountain Spotted fever can be very serious or even fatal without early intervention.[45]

west nile virus – transmitted by mosquitos. Symptoms: fever, headache, body aches, fatigue, rash, swollen lymph, inflammation of brain or membrane surrounding brain and spinal cord.

XII. THE COMMON DENOMINATOR IN CHRONIC FATIGUE & FIBROMYALGIA

It is believed by many that Florence Nightingale, Charles Darwin, Alfred Nobel and Job suffered from symptoms we know of today as CFS & Fibromyalgia. What would be the common denominator between then and now, over that much time? I think viruses.

Without cell mediated immunity, the immune system produces antibodies to defend itself. The end result is pain, inflammation and adverse effects on the central nervous system.

Upon testing, our chronic fatigue and fibromyalgia patients were found to be making abnormally high amounts of antibodies to three or more of the viruses discussed. It seems entirely possible that a viral infection causing inflammation would set the stage for other sensitivities such as, foods, chemicals, and molds. It may take multiple toxins and microorganisms before the body is compromised to the point where a person begins to suffer from chronic pain and fatigue and experience multiple chemical sensitivities.

After ruling out insect transmitted diseases and other pathophysiology mimicking CFS/FM, and reviewing lab reports of overproduction of antibodies to viruses, mold, chemicals, additives, preservatives and foods – and reviewing symptoms of CFS/FM – the common denominator among all the patients is the excessive antibody production to viruses. We know that many of these viruses are common childhood viruses to which we have all been exposed and that they stay with you for life. Viral sickness for a child is usually uneventful as it typically involves one or two viruses at a time. Reactivation in an adult can be quite a different story as it may activate some or all of these viruses at the same time - leading to long lasting fatigue and unexplained pain.

We like to talk about remission. Since these viruses stay with us for life, it would be of interest to put these viruses back into a dormant state. By doing this, it would decrease the load on an overwhelmed immune system; reduce damaging inflammation, thereby allowing the repair process to begin; restore metabolic pathways and allow the body to heal itself so that we can get back to living our lives.

Many of our patients refuse prescription drugs for a variety of reasons, some having to due with side-effects and costs. Given this, we created an all natural protocol. We believe that the symptoms of chronic fatigue and fibromyalgia have an underlying, chronic, viral component. Since 2009, we have been making the following recommendations to our patients and have had enough success that now we would like to share it with you.

After an extended visit with Mrs. Jones, we watch her as she leaves the clinic and makes her way to the car. The car door closes behind her and she gets on the cell phone to make a call. Simultaneously, the clinic phone rings. It's Mrs Jones.

From the clinic, *"Hi, are you ok?"*

"Oh, yes. I am so sorry to bother you, again, but my brain fog is so bad I can't remember anything you said!"

> You suffer from pain & fatigue.
> No one believes you.
> Your symptoms are invisible.
> You are in a battle.
> You need a plan.
> We have one.

We named it **FIBROBUSTERS®**.
The protocol is based on a natural anti-viral approach in order to overcome adverse symptoms caused by chronic hidden viruses.

XIII. **FIBROBUSTERS**® PROTOCOL

FIBROBUSTERS® is a natural anti-viral approach designed in the clinic to overcome adverse symptoms caused by chronic hidden viruses. First, we need to heal the gut. Restore function to the gut and you restore your immune system. This will take the load off an overwhelmed immune system and in addition, begin to restore metabolic pathways. It is then that the body can begin to heal itself. Let's begin:

Mineral concentrations of soils vary greatly throughout regions of the world. We suffer from mineral deplete farm soils. This translates directly to plant nutrient concentrations and the foods we eat.[56]

1. Choose a Natural Multi-Mineral supplement complete with naturally occurring organic acids.

As stated by EG Heinrich, "a complete spectrum of minerals" contains at least 70 minerals. This large number of minerals has to include many of the "rare earth" minerals. These rare earth minerals are necessary, in addition to the more commonly known minerals. A "complete spectrum of minerals" lowers pH thereby inhibiting bacterial and viral replication. Cellular fluids function properly only because of a carefully maintained ratio of minerals in conjunction with vitamins. The interaction of the two enables the body cells to take in nutrients and dispose of toxins that are the by-products of that metabolism.

A lack of minerals inhibits detoxification. Detoxifying occurs whenever the body begins to expel and eliminate anything that causes the body to make antibodies. This process occurs naturally, but if you lack minerals, it will not be complete. A balanced immune system depends on a clean detoxed body and this can only be obtained through the elimination of waste. Detox through optimal cellular metabolism with a complete spectrum of at least 70 minerals makes an incredible difference.[63]

As well, many minerals and their naturally occurring organic acids are removed from water to make way for chlorine and flouride. According to the European Agency for the Evaluation of Medicinal Products, "Humic acid is part of the human diet as they are contained in drinking water."[62]

Minerals are necessary for the function of vitamins, proteins, carbohydrates, fats, enzymes and in making RNA and DNA. There are many mineral supplements to choose from. We made Virasyl® for our patients. It is a rich multi mineral supplement that contains its own naturally occurring organic acids of humic and fulvic acid. Research indicates that these organic acids have natural anti-viral, anti-inflammatory properties, and mast cell protecting effects, associated with their function.[59, 60, 61]

2. Foods to avoid if you are suffering from chronic viruses that may be contributing to the cause of pain & fatigue: **Avoid nuts** (including peanut butter). It is the amino acid l-arginine that we want to avoid as it tends to fuel a virus. Avoid ALL nuts for a while. If you decide to reintroduce them into your diet at a later time, go slow to see if you react. **Avoid citrus** fruits (this includes OJ, lemon water & tomato). Citrus fruits release histamine and tomatoes are high in histamine.

3. Drink only freshwater. Don't drink chlorine or flouride!

4. Avoid gluten (wheat products like bread & pasta) as it has been implicated in autoimmune disorders. The inability to digest gluten triggers inflammation in the gut, which then leads to destroyed membranes, followed by malabsorption of nutrients.[44]

5. Avoid artificial sweeteners. Try Stevia instead.

6. Avoid soft drinks. Substitute with sparkling water.

7. Take a B-complex supplement + B12 sublingual in the morning. High carbohydrate intake (typical American diet) and alcohol depletes all B vitamins. They need to be replaced.

8. Eat protein for breakfast. You'll feel better all day long.

9. Avoid hydrogenated oils of any kind as they are rigid and not found in nature. Every cell has two layers of lipid molecules. Your body will use the oils and fats that you consume to make these cellular membranes. It is essential at the cellular level, beginning with a healthy flexible cell wall, to bring in nutrients and excrete waste. Essential fatty acids are critical in order to make healthy cells.

10. Sleep is an immune response. You need to sleep. Try magnesium 200-400mg before bed.*
Turn off the lights! (TV, LED clocks, internet) Besides the eyes and pineal gland, all cells have particles that respond to light. They need to be recharged.

11. Low on Vitamin D? The mineral Boron is essential for absorption of Vitamin D, which is essential for absorption of calcium.[65] *Always check with your healthcare practitioner before taking any supplements.

12. Sweat!! Steam rooms, sauna, hot baths with sea salts.

ALTERNATIVE THERAPIES PROVEN EFFECTIVE:
1. Low level light laser. It is coherent, monochromatic and polarized allowing photons to reach the cells and be converted to biochemical energy enabling healing and pain relief for the soft tissues. Excellent for joint pain, muscle strain to neck and back, carpal tunnel syndrome and post herpetic neuralgia.[66]
2. Acupuncture or ETPS (needleless acupuncture) [46]

IN ADDITION:

A.) Watch out for anti-perspirants with aluminum. Think about it: this application is over glandular tissue with lymph nodes directly underneath.

B.) The application of soaps, lotions, perfumes and nail products add up over time. Try to find products free of parabens, sulfates, phthalates, toluene and formaldehyde.

C.) Be aware of GMO foods. Learn more about it at www.worldhealth.us [64]

D.) Forgive yourself. The emotional component tied to our state of health is most likely more important than anything else. Whatever it is, whatever happened, forgive yourself. Do this everyday.

E.) Classical music. It is healing. Try Vivaldi, Bach or Mozart. Albert Einstein who was enchanted by music once said, *"Mozart's music is so pure it seems to have been ever present in the universe."* [51]

Some patients reported feeling better within days and for others, it took a few months. As stated earlier, we found that patients with symptoms of chronic fatigue syndrome were making antibodies to the enterovirus family such as cocksackie A & B and echo viruses. For these patients it takes a much longer period of time to begin feeling better. Be patient. Healing takes time.

XIV. THE IMMUNE RESPONSE

As stated earlier, we come into contact with infectious pathogens daily. We are generally able to mount a defense as we are equipped with different types of immune responses.

Immune response begins with recognizing foreign material and then creating a reaction to get rid of it. This involves a variety of cells and the molecules they secrete. The extent of the immune system is vast and complex. The following is but a glimpse at the immune response, only addressing histamine and antibody production.

Mast cells are immune cells found in connective tissue and mucous membranes. They release inflammatory mediators such as prostaglandin, leukotrienes and histamine. These mediators promote vasodilation, increase vascular permeability, increase mucous secretions and cause fever. Mast cells are activated by complement fragments from IgG and IgM; and activated directly from IgE.

Of these inflammatory markers, for now, let's look closer at histamine.

HISTAMINE

Histamine is a neurotransmitter found abundantly in the central nervous system and functions as a signaling molecule in the gut, skin and for the immune system.

Histamine receptors (**H1-H4**) are located throughout the central nervous system, skin, gut and in the blood:

H1 receptors in mucosal linings, when activated, give rise to allergy symptoms like itchy, watery eyes, nasal congestion and hives.

H2 receptors in the stomach are regulated by the vagus nerve and release gastric acid. H2 blockers are widely prescribed for gastric disorders. Some antidepressants have H2 blocking effects; and as well, there are reports for efficacy of H2 blockers in schizophrenia.

In a journal article, *Histamine in the Nervous System*, Haas states, "Histamine released from mast cells, closely associated with immune response against gut microbes, plays a role in gastrointestinal infection, inflammation and tumor growth. Elevated levels of H1 and H2 are found in endoscopic biopsies from humans with food allergy and irritable bowel syndrome."[7]

Histamine is released from mast cells in an immune response to gut microbes of the wrong kind. But there are also foods that are high in histamine and foods that trigger a histamine response, such as tomatoes.

Histamine toxicity can present with symptoms such as: hives, itchy watery eyes, headache, stuffy nose, wheezing, shortness of breath, excess mucous, acid reflux, difficulty swallowing, coughing, stomach pain, cramping, diarrhea, confusion and dizziness.

The enzyme that degrades histamine in the gut is diamine oxidase (DAO). An article by Maintz and Novak discusses "histamine intolerance" because of impaired DAO activity in the gut.

H3 receptors inhibit histamine release and synthesis.

H4 receptors are found in tissues like blood, spleen, lung, liver and gut.

Histamine is a powerful neurotransmitter and signaling molecule that stimulates gastric acid, functions as a vaso-dilator, bronchoconstrictor and is involved in basic brain and body functions. Histamine plays a much bigger role in immune response than previously known. Haas states in a journal article, "The impact of histamine on neuroendo-crine control is well documented. Brain histamine is deep-ly concerned with the control of behavior, biological rhythms, body weight, energy metabolism, thermoregula-tion, fluid balance, stress and reproduction."[7]

Histamine is only active during wakeful hours and binds to NMDA receptors. So in theory, too much histamine over-stimulating NMDA receptors would cause over excitation of the central nervous system resulting in symptoms like stress and anxiety.

Mast cells (cells that secrete histamine) are activated by complement fragments from IgM and IgG; and directly from IgE or the antigen itself.

ANTIBODY PRODUCTION IS AN IMMUNE RESPONSE
Hypersensitivity reactions are measured by antibody production. The outcome can range from mild discomfort to irreversible tissue damage and autoimmune disorders.

The antibody (IgG) testing of viruses and the environmental panel, performed for our patients, is reflective of Type II or Type III hypersensitivities explained below.

Below is a brief review of all 4 types of hypersensitivities as measured by the production of antibodies:

Type I (IgE)
A relatively **immediate** reaction, happening within an hour or so, therefore it will likely be more obvious as to what caused the reaction, for example if you just cut the lawn and start wheezing soon after, then this is a "Type I" response. It is the mast cells unleashing histamines that take center stage in this act as they are responsible for in-

flammation, dilation of blood vessels and typical allergy responses such as: itchy, watery eyes, nasal congestion, sneezing, wheezing, asthma and anaphylaxis.

Type II (IgM/IgG)

(IgM indicates acute infection;

IgG indicates chronic infection)

Type II is a *delayed response* of the immune system caused by an antigen attached to a cell membrane. Therefore, this is **attached to the outside the cell**. The antigen presence creates an antibody that activates complement, causing injury to cells and tissue.

Cause: viruses, bacteria, molds, metals, additives, preservatives, chemicals, foods.

Reaction time: minutes to hours.

Manifestation: muscle & joint pain, headache, migraine, fever, fatigue, rash, canker sores, IBS, gastroenteritis, acid reflux, unexplained chest pain, shortness of breath, anxiety depression, brain fog, sleep disorders, Goodpasture's nephritis.

Typical treatment: anti-inflammatory and immunosuppressive agents.

WHAT IS AN ANTIBODY?

Take a second look at the front cover; the "Y" shaped objects are antibodies surrounding the foreign green antigen. Antibody production is part of a normal immune response to defend against harmful invaders such as viruses, bacteria, mold, or anything the body does not recognize.

Antibodies activating complement cause further damage to cells and tissues.

Antibody production does not control an infection.
It is an immune response that is termed, "Hypersensitity Reaction"in immunology.[57]

WHAT IS COMPLEMENT?

Complement is a group of proteins found in the serum that "complement" the immune system by assisting antibodies to clear the pathogen from the host, resulting in damage to tissues. Antibodies activate complement.

Complement fragments stimulate mast cells, which release inflammatory markers such as histamine, leukotrienes and prostaglandins.

Type III (IgM/IgG)

Type III is a *delayed response* caused by **floating** immune complexes (**antigen + antibody**, i.e; virus + antibody), in the blood that are trying to make their way out of the body, but instead becomes lodged in tissue causing intense inflammation. This "immune complex," can become stuck in tissue on its way out. Further activation of complement will cause even more tissue injury. Diseases from the immune complex are fairly common.

Cause: most likely microorganisms such as viruses, bacteria, molds, parasites.

Manifestation: systemic lupus erythematosus, kidneys (lupus nephritis), lungs, blood vessels, joints (rheumatoid arthritis), Arthus reaction, Farmer's lung disease.

Reaction time: up to 10 hours.

Typical treatment: anti-inflammatory agents.

Type IV

A *cell mediated* reaction, meaning that there is *no antibody production*; rather, the T-cell must migrate to the site of the antigen - as the antigen is **inside the cell**. This takes longer than an antibody response.

Reaction time: 2-7 days.

Example of causes: skin rash from nickel, chemicals, poison ivy, bacteria.

XV. VIRUSES – A CLOSER LOOK

Viruses exist everywhere. They are by far the most abundant parasites (organism living off of host) on the planet. The host range is broad to include: water, marine life, soil, plants, bacteria, fungus, insect, animals and humans.

Different viruses produce different clinical pictures. In addition, a given subtype of a virus can cause a variety of manifestations in different hosts.

The following gives a little more information on common viruses for which we tested, to include herpes 1-6, Parvo B-19, Enteroviruses, and Adenovirus.

HERPES
Herpes viruses infect most of the human population and persons living past middle age usually have antibodies to most of the herpes viruses 1 - 6. Herpes viruses are a leading cause of human viral disease, second only to influenza and cold viruses. They are capable of causing observable disease, like chicken pox, or remaining silent for many years only to be reactivated later in life, such as shingles.

77

The name herpes comes from the Latin *herpes* which, in turn, comes from the Greek word *herpein* which means "to creep." This reflects the creeping or spreading nature of the skin lesions caused by many herpes virus types. So far, herpes 7 and 8 have also been discovered. Herpes 7 is much like herpes 6; and Herpes 8 can be found in the biopsy of a Kaposi's sarcoma. As viruses continue to mutate, it may not end here at 8.

HERPES 1&2

Primary infection occurs through a break in the mucus membranes of the mouth or throat, via the eye or genitals or directly via minor abrasions in the skin. The hallmark of herpes infection is the ability to infect epithelial mucosal cells or lymphocytes. Once the virus has passed a point of entry, it then travels up a nerve to the CNS where it may stay for years, followed by potential reactivation years later. Reactivation may occur due to various events such as injury, stress or hormone imbalance. With reactivation, the virus travels back down the nerve to the surface of the body, causing tissue damage.

Most individuals are infected during childhood; initial infection usually goes unnoticed, although minor blisters may form. Symptoms of an outbreak such as blisters, pain, inflammation, redness, swollen lymph nodes and fever are a result of a responding immune system.[14] The production of antibodies alone will not be able to control the infection.

Once you are infected with herpes, it's with you for life. Although painful, most repeat infections resolve on their own. More serious infections involving the eye are due to ulceration of the cornea. Repeated infections can lead to blindness. Infections involving the central nervous system causing meningitis and encephalitis are rare, but often fatal.

Herpes-1: Primarily associated with cold sores around the mouth and sometimes lesions around the eye.

Herpes-2: Primarily associated with genital and anal lesions. This infection has been increasing in incidence and prevalence every year. More than 45 million people in the USA are currently infected with herpes-2, and more than a million new cases are diagnosed annually. Herpes 2 is the most common sexually transmitted disease in the world.[1]

HERPES & ALZHEIMER'S?

Alzheimer's disease affects 10% of people over age 65 and 20% of those over age 75. In the UK, this amounts to about 750,000 cases, and around 4 million in the USA. A particular version (allele) of the human ApoE4 gene is known to be a risk factor for the development of Alzheimer's disease, but by no means do all of those who carry this version get Alzheimer's.

According to the Journal of Pathology from Manchester, UK, "The brains of Alzheimer's disease sufferers are characterized by amyloid plaques and neurofibrillary tangles." Herpes simplex virus type 1 is a strong risk factor for Alzheimer's when it is in the presence of the components that make the amyloid plaques in the brain. We discovered a striking localization of herpes simplex virus type 1 DNA within plaques: in Alzheimer's diseased brains, 90% of the plaques contained the viral DNA." [12]

A large proportion of elderly people have herpes simplex virus in their brains, whether or not they have Alzheimer's disease. Could HSV infection and the ApoE4 gene combined play a role in Alzheimer's disease? [10, 11]

Is it possible that this viral infection would allow activation of the genetic component causing Alzheimer's?

HERPES 3
Varicella *(Chicken pox)* Chicken pox is very contagious as it is spread through air droplets or from direct contact with the rash. Infection normally occurs in childhood. The virus can spread into the bloodstream. Complications are rare, but may include CNS infection.[9] The following are afflictions known to be caused by a herpes 3 infection; all affecting the nervous system:
Shingles, Ramsay Hunt syndrome, and Bell's palsy.

Zoster (Shingles) Shingles occurs in people who have had chickenpox and represents a reactivation of the dormant varicella-zoster virus. Zoster means "girdle" as it tends to form a rash around the thorax like a belt in many patients. This linear rash follows the dermatome (area of skin innervated by single spinal nerve). Zoster is the most serious when cranial nerves are involved, causing diseases such as *Ramsay Hunt Syndrome, Bell's palsy* and inflammatory eye disorders.

Ramsay Hunt syndrome type I, is caused by the spread of the varicella-zoster virus to facial nerves and is characterized by intense ear pain, a rash around the ear, mouth, face, neck, and scalp, and paralysis of facial nerves. Other symptoms may include hearing loss, vertigo (abnormal sensation of movement), and tinnitus (abnormal sounds). Taste loss in the tongue and dry mouth and eyes may also occur. Some cases of Ramsay Hunt syndrome type I do not require treatment. When treatment is needed, medications such as antiviral drugs or corticosteroids may be prescribed. Vertigo may be treated with the drug diazepam. Generally, the outcome of Ramsay Hunt syndrome type I is quite favorable; however, in some cases, hearing loss may be permanent, vertigo may last for days or weeks and facial paralysis may be temporary or permanent.[13]

Bell's Palsy is the spread of the virus to cranial nerve VII (facial nerve). This nerve disorder afflicts approximately 40,000 Americans each year. It can strike almost anyone at any age; however, pregnant women and people who have diabetes, influenza, a cold, or some other upper respiratory ailment are more predisposed to an attack. In addition to one-sided facial paralysis along with a possible inability to close the eye, symptoms of Bell's palsy may include pain, tearing, drooling, hypersensitivity to sound in the affected ear, and impairment of taste.

There is no specific treatment for Bell's palsy. Treatment is usually aimed at protecting the eye from drying at nighttime. Some physicians may prescribe a corticosteroid drug to help reduce inflammation and an analgesic to relieve pain. The prognosis for Bell's palsy is generally very good. With or without treatment, most patients begin to get significantly better within a couple of weeks, and approximately 80% recover completely within 3 months. For some, however, the symptoms may last longer. In a few cases, the symptoms may never completely disappear.[13, 14]

Reactivation via cranial nerve V (Trigeminal) can affect the eye causing uveitis, keratitis, conjunctivitis, paralysis of muscles that move the eye, and iritis.[13]

Well after many of the symptoms have resolved from a zoster attack, the nerve pain can linger, referred to as "post herpetic neuralgia," along with increased sensitivity to touch of the skin, referred to as "hyperesthesia."[13]

HERPES 4

Herpes 4 is **Epstein Barr** virus, aka, mononucleosis, or "The Kissing Disease." There is a well established relationship between herpes 4 and Burkitt's lymphoma in Africa; nasopharyngeal carcinoma in the orient; and infectious mononucleosis in the west. It was first discovered as the causative agent of Burkitt's lymphoma and it was later found that patients with infectious mononucleosis have antibodies that react with Burkitt's lymphoma cells.[2] Infection is also associated with B cell lymphomas in patients with an inactive immune system, certain T cell lymphomas, and Hodgkin's disease.[9]

Disease:	Comments:
Infectious mononucleosis	Primary infection resolves on its own.
Burkitt's lymphoma	Cells contain latent virus.
Hodgkin's disease	Sporadic lymphoma; latent virus found in approx. 50% of cases.
Nasopharyngeal carcinoma	Malignant squamous epithelial tumor of the nasopharynx; Cells contain latent virus.
Oral hairy leukoplakia	Viral replication on top of the tongue. Affects mostly HIV+ individuals.

A large proportion of the population (90-95%) is infected with Epstein-Barr virus; as well, these people, although usually asymptomatic, will shed the virus from time to time throughout life. Up to 80% of students entering college in the US are seropositive for the virus and many of those that are negative will become positive while at college.[14]

HERPES 5

Herpes 5 is **Cytomegalovirus (CMV)**. It is the largest, therefore "mega," of the herpes viruses. Cytomegalovirus infection is found in a significant proportion of the population. By college age, about 15% of the US population is infected and this rises to about half by 35 years of age. The virus is spread in most secretions, particularly saliva, urine, vaginal secretions and semen (which has the highest titer of any body fluid). These finding indicate that *cytomegalovirus is also sexually transmitted.*[14]

Antibody production (IgG) is an immune response to chronic infection, however it will not be able to control the infection.[14] The symptoms of CMV infection are similar to those of mononucleosis: fatigue, general discomfort, uneasiness, or ill feeling (malaise), joint stiffness, loss of appetite, muscle aches or joint pain, night sweats, prolonged fever, sore throat swelling of the lymph nodes, weakness, weight loss. In immune compromised people, CMV can attack specific organs: eyes, lungs, GI tract, brain.[15]

The following table shows the organs where CMV may reside and the major symptoms of chronic infection:

ORGAN INFECTED WITH CMV	MAJOR SYMPTOMS
Eye	Blindness, floaters, visual impairment
Lungs	Pneumonia
GI tract	Difficulty swallowing, ulcers, diarrhea
Brain	Coma, encephalitis, seizures

Several antiviral medications are available to treat CMV. These medicines require close monitoring for side effects. Antiviral drugs can help stop the virus from copying itself within the body. However, the drugs do not eliminate the virus from the body.

85

HERPES 6

Herpes 6 is found mainly in saliva. It infects almost all children by the age of two and stays for a lifetime. It replicates in B and T lymphocytes, megakaryocytes, glioblastoma cell and in the oropharynx. It can set up a hidden infection in T cells which may be activated later when the cells are set to divide. Infected cells are larger than normal with inclusions in both cytoplasm and nucleus. Cell-mediated immunity is essential for control of this virus. Antibody production does not control this infection.

Herpes 6 is also known as "roseola infantum" or **"sixth disease."** Antibody titers are highest in children and decline with age. Consequences of childhood infection appear to be mild. This is a common disease of young children and symptoms include fever, then rash on the trunk and sometimes upper respiratory tract infection with swollen glands. In adults, primary infection is associated with mononucleosis. Primary infections of adults are rare but have more severe consequences.[1] In adults, primary infection with HHV-6 can produce a mononucleosis-like illness and, more rarely, a severe disease, including encephalitis, myocarditis and myelosuppression.[16]

Herpes 6 has been associated with a number of neurological disorders, including encephalitis and seizures. It has been claimed to play a role in multiple sclerosis and chronic fatigue immunodeficiency syndrome.[9, 14]

Human Herpesvirus-6 and Its Effect on the GABA/Glutamate Balance in the Cerebrospinal Fluid and in the Brain From Patients With Epilepsy

A clinical trial sponsored by: National Institute of Neurological Disorders and Stroke (NINDS)

June 2004 "This study explores whether the human herpes virus-6 is associated with epileptic seizures. The virus may be involved in brain scarring, called mesial temporal sclerosis, which is seen in some epilepsy patients. The virus is also thought possibly to interfere with neurotransmitters - chemicals that brain cells use to communicate with each other. This study measured levels of two of these chemicals, GABA and glutamate, which are believed to play a role in the development of seizures. [11]

PARVOVIRUS B-19

Parvoviruses are among the smallest. There are now more than 50 parvoviruses that have been identified. Human parvovirus infections were only recognized in the 1980's. The best known human Parvovirus is referred to as **B19**. B-19 tends to infect rapidly dividing tissues, most commonly: the fetus, the intestinal epithelium, and red blood cell precursors.[9, 14]

First discovered in 1974, it wasn't until 1981 that it was associated with aplastic crisis in children. This event involves an acute depression in the production of red blood cells from the bone marrow where infection of the reticulocytes occurs. This event is short-lived and is usually not of great clinical significance except in patients with other hematological disorders such as sickle-cell anemia. This is followed by a rubella-like rash, which is usually the most obvious symptom of a B-19 infection.

Children are much more likely than adults to develop the rash. B-19 is also called *"erythema infectiosum"* or *"slapped cheek disease"*, because of the rash on the cheeks. It is also referred to as *"fifth disease"* because it was the fifth of a series of rashes, ordered in the sequence that they were reported, that all look very similar. The others are: measles (Rubeola), scarlet fever (Scarlatina), German measles (3-day measles, rubella) and Dukes' disease.

Most people are infected early in life and develop immunity; however adults can be infected as well. Adults may not manifest any symptoms at all, but they may develop the typical rash. This can be accompanied by swelling of the joints on both sides of the body which usually subsides in a few weeks, though the swelling can persist longer. This temporary arthritis like joint involvement happens in approximately 80% of patients.[14]

In approximately 5% of maternal B-19 infections occurring in the first half of the pregnancy, the mother may develop a serious anemia that may result in miscarriage.[14] If the virus crosses the placenta, it may replicate in erythroid cells of the fetus causing fetal anemia and non-immune hydrops fetalis (NIHF). Hydrops usually occurs about 4 weeks after maternal infection.

"My Dog Has Parvo! Did I get it from my Dog?"
The human parvovirus B-19 is different from the parvoviruses which cause problems in dogs and cats. In dogs, it is called canine parvovirus which can cause severe disease. Feline panleukopenia in cats is caused by feline parvovirus and can cause death as a result of destroyed immune system. Vaccines against both of these are available.

ADENOVIRUS
Adenoviruses are frequently the cause of acute upper respiratory tract infections typically presenting as a cold, sore throat and/or tonsillitis. This virus primarily attacks tissues

of the inner surface of the eyelid, respiratory tract, gut and genitourinary tracts.

ADENOVIRUS SYNDROMES	SYMPTOMS
Upper respiratory infection	runny nose, sore throat, tonsillitis, fever
Pharyngo-conjunctival fever	Fever, conjunctivitis, sore throat, headache, rash, swollen lymph nodes
Lower respiratory infection	Bronchitis, pneumonia, fever, cough
Pneumonia	Fever, respiratory distress, cough; severe in children and infants
Pertussis-like Syndrome	Fever, cough attack, post-tussive vomiting
Acute Respiratory Disease	bronchitis, pneumonia, fever
Keratoconjunctivitis	Headache, conjunctivitis followed by inflammation of cornea, swollen lymph nodes in neck
Acute follicular/ Hemor-rhagic conjunctivitis	swelling around cornea, subconjunctival hemor-rhage, swollen lymph nodes in neck
Acute Hemorrhagic cystitis	Blood in urine, fever, painful urination
Gastro-enteritis	Diarrhea (especially in children <4 years old) low grade fever

Rare results of adenovirus infections include: meningitis, encephalitis, arthritis, skin rash, myocarditis, pericarditis, hepatitis.[14]

PICORNAVIRUSES

Picornaviruses are among the most diverse (more than 200 serotypes) and oldest known viruses.[1] Picornavirus family includes 9 genera[1]:

AFFECTS HUMANS	AFFECTS ANIMALS
Enteroviruses: Polio Echo Coxsackie A&B	*Cardiovirus* (mainly found in rodents)
Parechovirus (formerly echo 22 & 23)	*Aphthovirus* (foot & mouth disease)
Rhinovirus (common cold)	*Erbovirus* (equine rhinitis B)
Hepatitis A (hepatitis in humans)	*Teschovirus* (mainly found in pigs)
Kobuvirus (affects cattle and swine)	

The Picornavirus family causes a wider range of illnesses than other virus families. Infection by different picornaviruses may happen without ever knowing it, or it may cause meningitis and/or encephalitis; appear as the common cold; present with fever/rash illnesses such as, hand-foot-and-mouth disease; herpangina (mouth blisters); inflammation of muscles, testes, heart, heart lining, eyelids and or liver (hepatitis).[2]

ENTEROVIRUSES
Widely known because of polio, enteroviruses have several subgroups:
3 serotypes of Polio
23 serotypes of group Coxsackie A
6 serotypes of group Coxsackie B
> 31 serotypes of Echo.

Enterovirus infections are common in humans; seasonal peak is in autumn; many infections are frequently undiagnosed.[2] Most patients infected with an enterovirus remain without symptoms; but in small children fevers caused by unidentified enteroviruses are relatively common and sometimes accompanied by a rash.

DISEASE FROM ENTEROVIRUSES	POLIO	COXSACKIE A	COXSACKIE B	ECHO
Meningitis	yes	yes	yes	yes
Acute Respiratory Distress	no	yes	yes	yes
Paralysis	yes	yes	yes	yes
Fever with rash	no	yes	yes	yes
Myocarditis	no	yes	yes	no
Orchitis	no	no	yes	yes

SYSTEMIC INFECTION CAUSED BY ENTEROVIRUS:

Central Nervous system: encephalitis.

Heart: mostly from coxsackie B; myocarditis, pericarditis.

Skeletal muscle: "Myalgic encephalomyelitis" – currently labeled a syndrome, there are few if any physical signs however there are many symptoms. The most prominent symptom is fatigue from even minor physical activity and presents along with psychological depression.[1]

Skin and mucous membranes: mostly from coxsackie A – rash with other symptoms.[3]

The ingested virus replicates in tissues of the throat or gut. The ingested viruses infect cells of the back of the throat and tonsils where they replicate and shed into the alimentary tract. From here they have access to pass further down the gastrointestinal tract. This virus remains stable in an acid environment and therefore is able to survive beyond the stomach, passing into the intestine to set up further infections in the intestinal mucosa. The virus also infects the lymphoid tissue (Peyer's patches) that are found in the lining of the gut.[2] Enterovirus replication can be observed in lymphoid tissue of the small intestine within 24-72 hours of ingestion of the virus.[3]

After multiplication in submucosal lymphatic tissues, enteroviruses pass to regional lymph nodes and give rise to a minor viremia (virus in the blood) that is transient and usually undetectable. During this low-grade viremia, the virus can spread to the liver, spleen, bone marrow, distant lymph nodes.[3]

Most enteroviruses in children are without symptoms; however, aseptic meningitis in infants is the most common display of enterovirus, while myocarditis (inflammation of the heart) and pleurodynia (pain in chest) are the most common symptoms of enterovirus in adolescents and young adults.[1]

The overall incidence of Picornavirus infections is unknown, as everyone around the globe is susceptable.[3]

XVI. THE FUTURE OF VIRUSES

In an article by Curtis Suttle, he states, "Each infection has the potential to introduce new genetic information into an organism or progeny virus, thereby driving the evolution of both host and viral assemblages. Probing this vast reservoir of genetic and biological diversity continues to yield exciting discoveries."[55]

Viruses with the the ability to cause disease could also be of concern if used as a biological weapon.

On the other hand, they are of high value when assisting us in understanding molecular genetics because of their usefulness in transferring genes into a cell of interest. It looks entirely promising that viruses could be a method of delivery for cancer treatments and gene therapy in the near future.[55]

Our understanding of viruses in the global system continues to unfold before us as we move forward in life sciences and medicine.

In the meantime, if we are to be the host, let them lie dormant!

GLOSSARY

adenovirus - originally "adenoid degenerative virus" or "adenoid-pharyngeal conjuctival virus."[2]

alimentary canal - the mucous membrane "long tube" of the digestive system. It is the canal through which food passes and waste is eliminated.

antibody - a protein molecule formation provoked by the immune system in defense to an antigen. All antibodies are immune globulins (IgG, IgM, IgE, IgA).

antigen - any substance which the body sees as foreign and consequently stimulates a defense against it by the production of antibodies.

carditis - inflammation of the heart.

coxsackie virus - from the name of a town along the Hudson River south of Albany, NY, where the virus was first recognized in 1898.[2]

cytomegalovirus - from the Greek *kytos*, "cell" = *mega*, "huge"; so called because cells infected by this virus become notably swollen. Human herpes virus 5.[2]

cytopathic - that kills cells.[1]

echo virus - ECHO an acronym for, "Enteric Cytopathic Human Orphan". So named because when discovered they were bereft of associated diseases.[2]

ELISA - enzyme-linked immunoassorbent assay.[1]

epithelial - tissue that covers the whole surface of the body. These cells are packed together in one or more layers.

GABA - gamma aminobutyric acid, an inhibitory neurotransmitter in the central nervous system.

herpes - is a borrowing of the Greek word that appears in Hippocratic writing as a term for a spreading cutaneous eruption. The root word is the Greek *herpein*, "to creep." The Latin equivalent *is serpere*, "to crawl, to move or spread slowly." To the Romans a *serpens* was a creeping thing, a snake,. The Greek zoster denotes a girdle. Hence, herpes zoster is an eruption that tends to creep around the torso. But it is only half a girdle" because the eruption of herpes zoster almost never crosses the midline from one side to the other. A common term for the disease is shingles, a term hobson-jobsoned from the Latin *cingulum*, "a girdle." Herpes simplex (Latin simplex, "simple or plain") is the name given to a virus that occurs in two types. Type 1 causes ordinary "cold sores, " such as erupt around the mouth, sometimes in response to fever. Type 2 causes recalcitrant genital sores that are anything but simple for the sufferer.[2]

humoral - pertaining to the humors, or certain fluids, of the body.[1]

IgG antibodies - IgG is the most abundant of the circulating antibodies. It readily crosses the walls of blood vessels and enters tissue fluids. IgG also crosses the placenta and confers passive immunity from the mother to the fetus. IgG protects against bacteria, viruses, and toxins circulating in the blood and lymph.[1]

IgM antibodies - IgMs are the first circulating antibodies to appear in response to an antigen. However, their concentration in the blood declines rapidly. This is diagnostically useful, because the presence of IgM usually indicates a current infection by the pathogen causing its formation. IgM consists of five Y-shaped monomers arranged in a pentamer structure. The numerous antigen-binding sites make it very effective in agglutinating antigens. IgM is too large to cross the placenta and hence does not confer maternal immunity.[1]

incidence - the number of cases of a disease, abnormality, accident, etc., arising in a defined population during a stated period, expressed as x cases per 1000 persons per year.[1]

inflammatory response - an immune reaction caused by the release of histamine, kinins and other chemical messengers that increase the permaeability of nearby capillaries, which causes redness and swelling of tissues.

limbic system - the emotional brain. Part of the brain that regulates behavior such as eating, drinking, aggression, sexual activity, and emotional expression.

lymphocyte - a white blood cell. Lymphocytes play a major role in both cellular and humoral immunity, and thus several different functional and morphologic types must be recognized, i.e. the small, large, B-, and T-lymphocytes, with further morphologic distinction being made among the B-lymphocytes.[1]

metabolic pathway - an orderly series of enzyme-mediated chemical reactions that lead to a final product.

myalgia - pain in the muscles.[1]

pineal gland - an endocrine gland located near the midline of the brain that produces melatonin, a hormone involved in biological rhythms.

rhinovirus - a virus typically causing an upper respiratory tract infection. From the Greek *rhinos*, "the nose."[2]

Sjögren's syndrome - a symptom complex of unknown etiology, usually occurring in middle-aged or older women, marked by the triad of keratoconjunctivitis sicca with or without lacrimal gland enlargement, xerostomia with or without salivary gland enlargement, and the presence of connective tissue disease, usually rheumatoid arthritis but sometimes systemic lupus erythematosus, scleroderma, or polymyositis. An abnormal immune response has been implicated.[1]

viremia - the presence of viruses in the blood, usually characterized by malaise, fever, and aching of the back and extremities.[1]

virus - any of a number of small, obligatory intracellular parasites with a single type of nucleic acid, either DNA or RNA. The nucleic acid is enclosed in a structure called a capsid, which is composed of repeating protein subunits called capsomeres, with or without a lipid envelope. The complete infectious virus particle, called a virion, must rely on the metabolism of the cell it infects. Viruses are morphologically heterogeneous, occurring as spherical, filamentous, polyhedral, or pleomorphic particles. They are classified by the host infected, the type of nucleic acid, the symmetry of the capsid, and the presence or absence of an envelope.[1]

REFERENCES

1. Holmin LR. Alfred Nobel. *J Clin Rheumatol 1996 Oct; 2 (5): 251-6.*

2. The Bible. Today's English Version. Job 6:7; 6:13-14; 7:3-4; 30:16-17; 17: 2-4.

3. Inanici F. Yunus MB. History of fibromyalgia: past to present. *Curr Pain Headache Rep.* Department of Medicine, University of Illinois College of Medicine, Peoria 2004 Oct;8(5):369-78.

4. Harris RE. *Chronic Pain and Fatigue Research Center.* U of Michigan

5. Harris ED. Budd RC. Genovese MC. Firestein GS. Sargent JS. Sledge CB. *Kelley's Textbook of Rheumatology.* 7th ed. St. Louis, MO: WB Saunders; 2005:525.

6. Rakel RE. Bope ET. *Conn's Current Therapy* 2008. 60th ed. Philadelphia, PA: Saunders Elsevier; 2008.

7. Haas HL. Sergeeva OA. et al; Histamine in the nervous system, Institute of Neurophysiology Heinrich-Heine-University Duesseldorf, Germany, *Physiology Review* 88: 1183-1241, 2008

8. Pathmicro.med.sc.edu/ghaffar/hyper00.htm; University of South Carolina School of Medicine, microbiology and immunology.

9. http://www.microbiologybytes.com

10. Itzhaki RF. et al. Herpes simplex virus 1 in brain and risk of alzheimer's disease *Lancet* 349: 241-244, 1997.

11. Dobson CB. Itzhaki RF. Herpes simplex virus type 1 and alzheimer's disease" *Neurobiology Aging* 20:457-465, 1999.

12. Wozniak MA, Mee AP, Itzhaki RF. Herpes simplex virus type 1 DNA is located within Alzheimer's disease amyloid plaques. *J Pathology.* 2009 Jan;217(1):131-8.

13. Gilden DH. Mahalingam R. et al, Herpesvirus infections of the nervous system. *Nat Clin Pract Neurology.* 2007 3: 82-94.

14. University of South Carolina University of Medicine- Microbiology and Immunology online.

15. www.nlm.nih.gov/cmv

16. Stoeckle M. Y. The spectrum of human herpesvirus 6 infection: from roseola infantum to adult disease; *Annual Review of Medicine* Vol. 51: 423-430 Feb 2000.

17. Cann A. http://www.microbiologybytes.com/virology/.

18. Holmes RL. Lutwick LI. Picornavirus overview emedicine.medscape.com/article/22543

19. Morimoto K. Fahnestock M. and Racine R J. Kindling and status epilepticus models of epilepsy: rewiring the brain. *Prog. Neurobiol.* 73, 1–60. 2004

20. Suzuki J. Investigations of epilepsy with a mutant animal (EL mouse) model. *Epilepsia* 45 (Suppl. 8), 2–5. 2004

21. Foldvary-Schaefer N. Wyllie E. Epilepsy. Goetz CG, ed. *Textbook of Clinical Neurology.* 3rd ed. Philadelphia, PA: Saunders Elsevier; ch.52. 2007

22. Malipiero U. Heuss C. Schlapbach R. Tschopp J. Gerber U. Fontana A. Involvement of the N-methyl-D-aspartate receptor in

neuronal cell death induced by cytotoxic T cell-derived secretory granules. *Eur. J. Immunol.* 29, 3053–3062. 1999

23. Getts M. T. Kim B. S. Miller S. D. Differential outcome of tolerance induction in naive versus activated Theiler's virus epitope-specific CD8+ cytotoxic T cells. *J. Virol.* 81, 6584–6593. 2007

24. Nair A. Hunzeker J. Bonneau R H. Modulation of microglia and CD8(+) T cell activation during the development of stress-induced herpes simplex virus type-1 encephalitis. *Brain Behav. Immun.* 21, 791–806. 2007

25. Hunsperger E A, Roehrig J T. Temporal analyses of the neuropathogenesis of a West Nile virus infection in mice. *J. Neurovirology.* 12, 129–139. 2006

26. Getts D R, et al. Viruses and the immune system: their roles in seizure cascade development *J Neurochem*, 2008 Mar; 104 (5): 1167-76

27. Hosoya M. Sato M. Honzumi K. Katayose M. Kawasaki Y. Sakuma H. Kato K. Shimada Y. Ishiko H. and Suzuki H. Association of nonpolio enteroviral infection in the central nervous system of children with febrile seizures. *Pediatrics* 107, E12. 2001

28. Toth C. Harder S. and Yager J. Neonatal herpes encephalitis: a case series and review of clinical presentation. *Can. J. Neurol. Sci.* 30, 36–40. 2003

29. Dagan R. Shahak E. Prolonged meningoencephalitis due to epstein–barr virus with favorable outcome in a young infant. *Infection* 21, 400–402. 1993

30. Bale J F Jr. Human cytomegalovirus infection and disorders of the nervous system. *Arch. Neurology* 41, 310–320. 1984

31. Hukin J. Farrell K. MacWilliam L. M. Colbourne M. Waida E. Tan R. Mroz L. Thomas E. Case-control study of primary human herpesvirus 6 infection in children with febrile seizures. *Pediatrics*. 101, E3. 1998

32. Source: http://www.physorg.com/print73573729.html

33. Barzilai O. Ram M. Viral infection can induce the production of autoantibodies. *Current Opinion in Rheumatology* 19(6):636-743. 2007

34. King MW. Serotonin. *The Medical Biochemistry Page*. Indiana University School of Medicine.
http://themedicalbiochemistrypage.org/nerves.html

35. Jaffe RM, Deuster PA. A Novel treatment for fibromyalgia improves clinical outcomes in a community-based Study. *Journal of Musculoskeletal Pain* Vol. 6(2) 1998.

36. Jaffe, R. M. www.elisaact.com

37. www.msnbc.msn.com/id/22258423/ns/health-skin_and_beauty/ 12/14/2007

38. www.newbeauty.com: one state's ban on mercury in mascara 12/17/2007

39. www.wndu.com/mmm/headlines/5900561.hmtl

40. www.newbeauty.com/dailybeautyentry.aspx?id=403

41. www.urmc.rochester.edu/news/story/index.cfm
Univeristy of Rochester Medical Center

42. Darbe et al. Concentrations of parabens in human breast tumors. *Journal of Applied Toxicology* (24), 5. 2004.

43. www.johnleemd.com

44. Fasano, A. Systemic autoimmune disorders in celiac disease. *Current Opinion in Gastroenterology*, 22(6):674-679. 2006

45. Center for Disease Control and Prevention www.cdc.gov/ticks/symptoms/html

46. Hocking B. www.acumedmedical.ca

47. Knight, D. MS, PA-C; Moser, S. MS, PA-C; A case of herpes encephalitis; *ADVANCE for Physician Assistants*; p16-17 July-Aug. 2009

48. Deitch, Edwin A; Role of the gut in multiple organ dysfunction syndrome. *UMDNJ Research.* www.umdnj.edu

49. T.S. Wiley, *Lights out sleep sugar and survival*, Pocket Books 2000

50. Boosting vaccine power. *Scientific American* p77. Oct 2009

51. Isaacson, W. *Einstein His Life And Universe*, Simon & Schuster 2007.

52. www.virasyl.com

53. Hadhazy, A. Think twice: how the gut's "second brain" influences mood and well-being. *Scientific American.* Feb 12, 2010.

54. Harvard Health Publications .The gut-brain connection. *Harvard Health Publications.*https://www.health.harvard.edu/healthbeat/the-gut-brain-connection.

55. Suttle, Curtis A. Marine viruses – major players in the global system. *Nature Reviews Microbiology* 5, 801-812 October 2007

56. Groff, J.L et al. *Advanced Nutrition and Human Metabolism* 1995.

57. Roitt Brostoff, Male. Immunology, 5th Edition, Mosby 2000.

58. Schmutzhard E. Viral infections of the CNS with special emphasis on herpes simplex infections. J. Neurol. 248, 469–477. 2001

59. Klocking, R et al. Antiviral properties of humic acids. *Experientia,* Vol 28 issue 5 607-8, May 1972.

60. Ghosal, S et al. Mast cell protecting effects of shilajit and its constituents. *Phytotherapy Research* 3 (6); 24-252, 1989.

61. GK Joone et al. An in vitro investigation of the anti-inflammatory properties of K humate. *Inflammation* Vol 28 No. 3 June 2004.

62. EMEA/RRL/554/99 – FINAL February 1999

63. EG Heinrich, *Root of All Dieases* 2000

64. www.worldhealth.us

65. Source: http://www.vitamindcouncil.org/about-vitamin-d/vitamin-d-cofactors/boron/

66. Chung H. Dai T. Sharma SK Huang YY, The nuts and bolts of low level laster light therapy. *Anuual Biomedical Engineering* 2012 Feb;40(2):516-33.

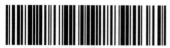

Made in the USA
Middletown, DE
24 December 2015